The Power of

CARBOHYDRATES,

PROTEINS, and LIPIDS

J. A. BITTENCOURT, Ph.D.

The Power of

CARBOHYDRATES,

PROTEINS, and LIPIDS

HOW TO MAKE WISE CHOICES IN DIET AND NUTRITION

FOURTH EDITION – 2018
Revised edition
(First Edition - 2011; Second Edition – 2012; Third Edition - 2015)

International Standard Book Number
ISBN-10: 1978372655
ISBN-13: 978-1978372658

Printed by CreateSpace, An Amazon.com Company
www.CreateSpace.com/ 7701743

Book available also at the website: www.amazon.com
E-mail: jabittencourt@hotmail.com

*D*edicated to everyone in search
of nutritional orientation
and optimum health.

PREFACE

For most people the selection of foods is related to a strong cultural tradition. However, not all culturally-acquired alimentary habits are healthy. Many people make their food choices based on habits acquired along their lifetime, according to food preferences and without any criteria really fundamental, and, sometimes, based on completely mistaken criteria.

Every day we make food choices that directly influence our health, well-being, and aging. Since choosing what to eat is the only *voluntary* step in the body's digestion and absorption processes, a knowledge of the biochemical processes related to food and its nutrients is essential for properly choosing what kind of food to eat. One of the meanings of the phrase "you are what you eat" is that to be healthy and fit you need to eat good food.

Through a scientific approach, based on the biological effects of food on the human body, this book presents updated nutritional information according to recent research and existing nutritional literature. The information presented here provides a basic nutritional knowledge that allows us to make wise choices relative to optimum nutrition.

Our knowledge of nutrition and how nutrients affect the body is constantly evolving through new data and research. Current nutritional science presents many well-defined tendencies regarding some matters that were controversial until a few years ago, like the phobia for foods that contain fats, developed over the last few decades, which made many people mistakenly avoid the ingestion of fats and excessively consume carbohydrates, particularly refined ones. The epidemic levels of obesity, diabetes, and cardiovascular diseases that have been observed in the developed countries over the last decades are due to lifestyle and modern diets, which are rich in sugars and refined foods, deprived of important nutrients.

The chapters of this book describe the biochemical properties and biological body functions of carbohydrates, proteins, and lipids, and their availability in foods. The role played by cholesterol and its possible influence on the promotion of cardiovascular diseases are discussed in detail. The importance of fibers, vitamins, minerals, antioxidant substances, and dietary supplements are also discussed.

The purpose of this book is *educational* and *informative* and is not intended as personal medical counseling. The information presented is also addressed to adults, not children, except when explicitly mentioned. Readers are advised to seek the orientation of a qualified health or nutrition professional before deciding to use any of the dietary supplements described in the book. The author and editor explicitly deny any responsibility, whatsoever, for any adverse effect that may result from the improper use of the information here presented.

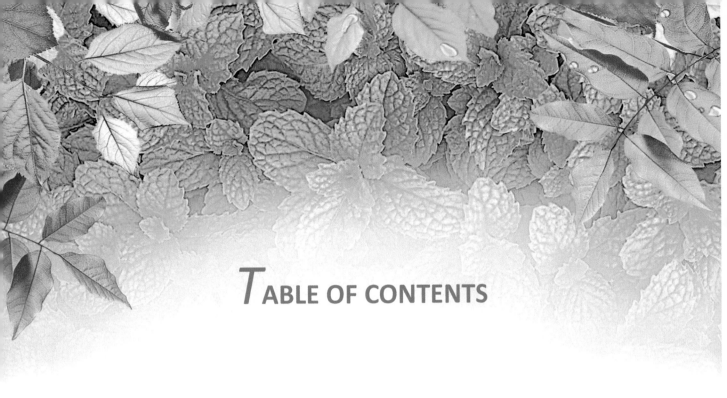

TABLE OF CONTENTS

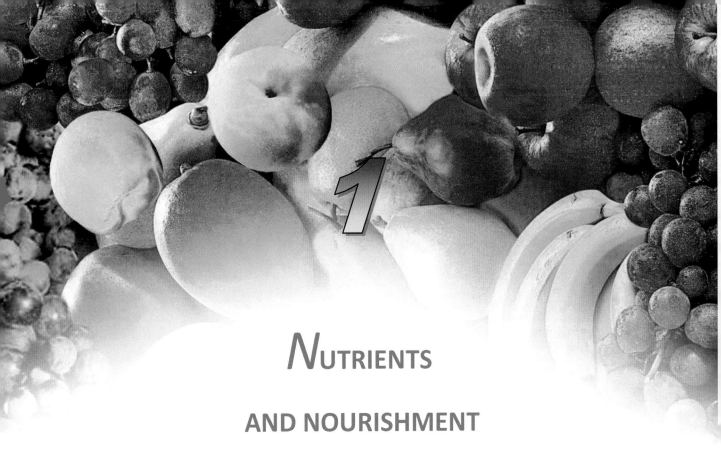

NUTRIENTS

AND NOURISHMENT

*O*ur body is a fantastic and highly complex *biochemical system*, constrained to well-defined genetic characteristics. Its healthy behavior depends directly on a wide variety of nutrients that must be obtained from food sources. Adequate nutrition is fundamental for a healthy metabolism, for normal growth and reproduction, for maintenance and operation of all body organs and tissues, for good physical activity, and for the immune system's ability to resist infections and diseases. Nutrition supplies the body with the biochemical energy and essential molecular constituents that are necessary for its healthy maintenance.

The term *nutrition* refers to the relationship between food, body health, and well-being. Optimal nutrition means that all necessary nutrients (as water, proteins, fats, carbohydrates, vitamins, minerals, and antioxidant substances) are supplied, in adequate amounts, by food, and used for the healthy operation of the body's biochemical processes. A proper knowledge of the various functions that the nutrients play in the body is fundamental to understand the importance of an optimized nutrition. The World Health Organization defines *health* as a state of total physical, mental, and social well-being, and not, merely, the absence of disease or illness. It also affirms that, to enjoy the best attainable health level, is a fundamental right of all human beings.

From a genetic point of view, each individual possesses its own biological and physiological characteristics and a unique body metabolism. Although each person may need about the same basic nutrients, some individual characteristics (i.e., genetic and physiological structure, physical activity levels, lifestyle, age, health condition, and nutrient absorption problems) may require the need for larger amounts of some nutrients. Nutritional deficiencies may result in disease, as when our food does not supply adequate amounts of the necessary nutrients for a balanced metabolism, as well as when it contains noxious substances, toxins, and antinutrients that interfere with the body's metabolism. Nutrition is science, and it is holistic by nature, since it affects the whole body.

> Our body is a highly complex biochemical system, constrained to individual genetic characteristics.

1.1 A MATTER OF CHOICE

*T*he only *voluntary* step in the control of the body's metabolism is the selection of foods for the alimentary (nourishment) diet. The nature and quality of the foods that we choose is important for good health. The *selection criteria* must consider not only the nutrients that a certain food contains, but also the absence of potentially harmful substances.

The development of pleasant, permanent, and healthy habits is a fundamental part of any plan for a lifetime of good health. Some *general principles* can guide us toward this objective. A positive self-image is important, besides determination, discipline, and self-responsibility, since good health cultivation depends primarily on personal decision. It is essential to have a basic knowledge of nutrition in order to be able to

> Health can be defined as a state of total physical, mental, and social well-being, and not, merely, the absence of disease or illness.

properly choose a diet with good levels of nutrients needed by the body. It is also important to live in a clean air environment, with appropriate sunlight exposure, good water quality, moderate physical exercise activities, and adequate rest periods.

Sometimes, small changes in diet and lifestyle habits can bring great health benefits, providing a more pleasant and long life, without depriving one of eating pleasure. Eating nutritious foods should be a celebration between nutritional science and eating pleasure, through which we are allowed to rationally choose the benefits of many foods and healthy nutrients, from our diet preferences. We don't have to be perfect in all our choices, avoiding all our favorite foods that may be potentially harmful, but should gradually move towards a diet and lifestyle that contribute to health improvement and that will allow the enjoyment of a better and longer life.

1.2 MACRONUTRIENTS

*E*veryday the body needs nutrients, substances that are absorbed by the body tissues to preserve health, supply energy, promote growth, recompose tissues, and restore the losses. Some substances, external to the body, are necessary in great amounts, being called *macronutrients*. There are basically four macronutrients that the body uses: water, carbohydrates, proteins, and lipids.

Before they can be used by the body tissues, the ingested foods need to be reduced to simpler components through *digestion* processes, which involve the action of *catalysts* (biochemical reaction-promoting substances) called *biological enzymes*. The simple products of digestion pass to the bloodstream by selective *absorption* processes in the intestinal tract.

> Eating nutritious foods should be a celebration between nutritional science and eating pleasure.

Water is the most abundant and main constituent of the body, representing about 55% of the total body mass. The blood is constituted of about 83% water, the kidneys 82%, the muscles 75%, the brain 74%, the liver 69%, and the bones 22%. Besides its hydrating function, water plays other important functions, such as the transport of water-soluble nutrients to all parts of the body and the elimination of residues and toxic products. The ingestion of about two to three liters of water per day is recommended. It is also important to certify that there are no harmful substances in the water, such as toxins and microorganisms. In a moderate climate, human beings can survive about five days without water.

The fluids present in the body (of which water is the main constituent) are distributed in two main compartments, separated by the cellular membrane: in the interior of cells, *intracellular* liquid, and outside the cells, *extracellular* liquid. The extracellular liquid is composed of the *interstitial* liquid (that externally bathes the cells) and the *blood plasma*. Each cell that constitutes the complex and organized set of tissues that form the body obtains its nutrients from the extracellular interstitial liquid in which it is submerged. This same liquid removes the metabolic degradation products eliminated by the cells.

> It is recommended the ingestion of about two to three liters of good quality water per day.

The normality of the interstitial fluid maintains the internal composition of the cells at a stable level, within narrow limits. The maintenance of the stability of this internal environment is called *homeostasis*. Homeostasis implicates a control of fluid composition and circulation, guaranteeing that each cell is immersed in a nutrient environment that is optimum for its function. Only limited variations of acid and alkaline substances, present in the circulating fluids (*acid-base balance*), are compatible with cellular health. The molecules that constitute the body and that maintain homeostasis come primarily from the metabolism of food molecules.

> The heart pumps blood through our body at a rate of about 100,000 times per day (about seventy times per minute).

The control of the composition and volume of body fluids, as well as the maintenance of a normal acid-base balance, depend mainly on the appropriate functioning of the lungs and kidneys, which interact among themselves and with all body cells through the blood. The circulation of liquids between the blood and other organs is continuous and maintained in a proper equilibrium. The heart pumps blood through the body at a rate of about 100,000 times per day (about seventy times per minute). All the blood passes through the kidneys, being filtered in those organs at a rate of about fifteen times every hour. A certain amount of water is eliminated daily, in the urine and through perspiration, needing replacement.

The *carbohydrates* from food act in the body as an energy source. They are present, for instance, in cereals (as rice, wheat, rye, barley, and malt), in products that contain flours (as breads, cakes, cookies, macaroni, and pasta), in tubers (as potato and manioc), in legumes (as beans, peas, soy, and peanut), in fruits and vegetables, and in all foods that contain sugars and starches. The carbohydrates ingested from food should be limited to an amount that allows the body to use all the glucose originating from carbohydrate metabolism, as well as the ingested fat, in order to avoid that any excess of both be stored in the body in the form of body fat. It will be explained in the chapter on carbohydrates that excess glucose entering the bloodstream, from carbohydrate metabolism, and that is not used for energy production, is reprocessed in the liver and metabolized into triglycerides (a type of fat), and stored as body fat.

> The carbohydrates from food act in our body as an energy source. Excess leads to body fat.

Proteins constitute the second most abundant substance in the body, after water, and are responsible for the formation and maintenance of body tissues and cells, which are being continually renewed. They form the enzymes (that catalyze the biochemical reactions in the body), the blood hemoglobin, the tissue collagen, and the defense antibodies. They perform countless important functions in the body. Proteins are present in meats, poultry, fish, eggs, milk, cheeses, beans, soy, peanuts, nuts, and seeds, and they are fundamental for proper nutrition. For basic body maintenance, it is usually recommended to ingest about 1g of high quality protein per

> Proteins are responsible for the formation and maintenance of body tissues and cells, and perform myriads of other important tasks.

kilogram of corporal weight, per day. For optimum protein levels, according to current specialists, this amount can be doubled, as long as the person has a normal renal function.

The *lipids* act in the body mainly in the formation of cellular membranes, nervous system tissues, brain tissues, and neurotransmitters, and can be used as a metabolic energy source. They are necessary for the transport of fat-soluble vitamins (A, D, E, and K) to the body cells, for the formation of sex hormones and the adrenal cortex, for maintaining body temperature, for forming a protective shield around muscles and nerves, and other important metabolic functions. Lipids are important constituents of food, mainly for supplying essential fatty acids (fundamental for good health) and for appropriate functioning of the brain and nervous system. They are present in nuts, seeds, peanuts, soy, vegetable grains, and foods of animal origin (meats, eggs, and cheeses). Different types of lipids in food accomplish different biochemical functions in the body. Ingestion should be selective and enough to supply the essential fatty acids the body requires.

> Lipids are necessary for the formation of cellular membranes, nervous system and brain tissues, and neurotransmitters.

The biochemical properties of carbohydrates, proteins, and lipids, and their metabolic functions in the body, are considered in detail in the next chapters. Alimentary *fibers* are usually present in many foods of vegetable origin, as whole grains, fruits, and vegetables. They are not digested by the body and they don't supply calories or energy. However, they are important constituents of our diet and contribute to regulate digestion, body metabolism, and good intestinal health.

1.3 VITAMINS, MINERALS, AND ANTIOXIDANTS

Besides the macronutrients, the body needs, in smaller quantities, a daily supply of other natural substances, *micronutrients* or *vitanutrients*, which include vitamins, minerals, and antioxidants, among others. Figure 1.1 shows the various types of nutrients and their main functions in the body.

Each *vitamin* and *mineral* plays a decisive role in one or more of the vital processes in the body's cells and tissues, acting mainly as controllers of metabolic processes. Vitamins are essential to good health. All vitamins are natural alimentary organic substances found in living beings, such as plants and animals. With a few exceptions, vitamins are considered *essential nutrients*. An essential vitanutrient is a substance necessary to promote good health and that cannot be produced by body metabolism, so that it must be obtained from food sources in appropriate amounts.

The functions that vitamins and minerals exert in human nutrition have been established along many years of clinical and biochemical research. Their important role in the activation of specific enzymes (substances that catalyze biochemical reactions in the body), and as antioxidant and cellular protecting agents, is already well recognized. Nowadays, more attention is focused on the therapeutic benefits of vitamins and minerals when ingested in doses well above the small amounts usually present in food or recommended for basic health maintenance.

> Vitamins are essential nutrients (with a few exceptions) that act as controllers of metabolic processes.

Many other substances that act together with vitamins and minerals for health maintenance, growth, and disease prevention have been identified. Those *antioxidant* substances, present in many fruits and colored vegetables, are usually called *phytochemical* substances (from the Greek *phyton*, which means "plant"), and they include *carotenoids*, *bioflavonoids*, and *polyphenols*.

1.4 ORTHOMOLECULAR SUBSTANCES

*T*he term *orthomolecular*, coined by the famous chemist and physicist Linus Pauling, Ph. D. (1901, USA - 1994), twice a Nobel Prize laureate, refers to substances (as vitamin C, for example) that are necessary for good health and life maintenance, and that are normally present in the human body. The term *orthomolecular medicine* was adopted by him to designate the preservation of good health and the treatment of physical and mental diseases through the use and diversification, in the human body, of orthomolecular substances. Orthomolecular nutrition is based on alimentary diets and supplements of essential vitamins, minerals, and other vitanutrients, specifically selected to promote good health and longevity. Substances as vitamin C and most of the other vitamins are notable for their low toxicity and absence of side effects, even when taken in quantities much larger than those usually available from food. The use of relatively large amounts of some vitamins, or megavitamin therapy, for the control of disease, to strengthen the immune system, to combat free radicals, and for the maintenance of a healthy organism is one of the important accomplishments of orthomolecular medicine. As affirmed by Linus Pauling, most medicines may eventually cause dangerous side effects, while vitamins and minerals are essential nutrients, basically inoffensive in their great majority, and necessary for life and good health maintenance.

Many phytochemical substances present in fruits and colored vegetables have antioxidant properties.

The molecule of most enzymes consists of a pure protein part, called *apoenzyme*, and a non-protein part, called *coenzyme*. Frequently, the coenzyme is a vitamin molecule or a molecule closely related to a vitamin. Therefore, many diseases caused by enzyme deficiency can be treated, or kept under control, through ingestion of large amounts of the vitamin that serves as coenzyme. Another example of orthomolecular therapy is the treatment of diabetes through insulin injections. Increase in vitamin C ingestion also reduces the need for insulin. Both vitamin C and insulin are constituents normally present in the body. Also, the immune system is strengthened by the ingestion of vitamins A, C, B_{12}, pantothenic acid, and folic acid. To produce most of the antioxidant enzymes, it is necessary to have appropriate levels of minerals like zinc, selenium, manganese, copper, and sulfur. Without enough of these necessary vitamins and minerals, the body cannot produce enough enzymes and, consequently, the free radicals (unstable substances, highly reactive and harmful to the body) take control, causing widespread damage to cells and tissues.

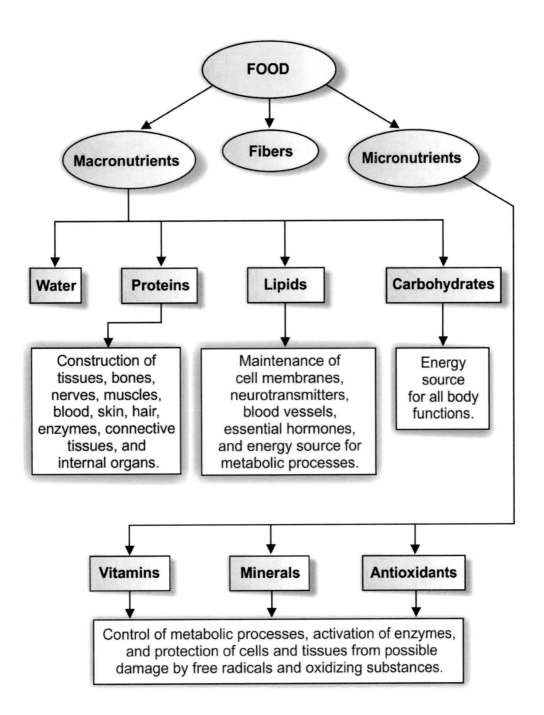

FIGURE 1.1 - Nutrients present in food and their main functions.

Other types of important nutrients that are also receiving increasing attention are the so-called *accessory alimentary factors*, substances that the body can produce in amounts that may be considered just appropriate for many people (if the necessary raw material is available), but not in levels considered optimum to promote good health. Everyone can need larger amounts of accessory alimentary factors, supplied through dietary supplements, for several reasons, either genetic or of health. The list of nutrients that possess great therapeutic value, when consumed in larger amounts than those supplied from a normal diet, for many individuals, it is one of the promising research areas in clinical nutrition. Examples of accessory nutrients include beta-carotene, bioflavonoids, lecithin, choline, garlic concentrates, fish oil, some fatty acids (as gamma-linolenic acid), and specific amino acids (as glutamine and carnitine).

> Orthomolecular nutrition is based on diets and natural supplements specifically selected to promote good health and longevity.

1.5 THE FOOD PYRAMID

*T*he recent nutritional literature has analyzed and criticized, based on current scientific evidence, the recommendations of the food guide pyramid built during the nineties by the US Department of Agriculture (USDA). This pyramid has in its base, or foundation, foods rich in carbohydrates (like breads, cakes, cereals, rice, pastas); in the inferior middle, mainly vegetables and fruits; in the superior middle, foods rich in proteins (such as meats, poultry, fish, eggs, beans, cheeses, and dairy products); and, at the top, foods rich in lipids (for sporadic use, with reservation). Virtually any food can be included in the USDA food guide pyramid. However, one of its basic problems is the lack of information regarding the different biochemical characteristics that exist between the various different types of carbohydrates, as well as between the various protein sources, and between the countless types of lipids and their effects (including hormonal ones) in the body.

Currently, some basic concepts contained in this pyramid (for instance, to eat more carbohydrates and less proteins, and to restrict the consumption of lipids) are being questioned, as a result of nutritional research and the epidemic levels of obesity, diabetes, and cardiovascular diseases that have been observed, along the last decades, in developed countries, as testified by current nutritional researchers. The main causes of modern diseases are linked to lifestyle and modern diets containing simple sugars and refined carbohydrates (in the form of cereals,

> The food guide pyramid lacks information regarding the different biochemical properties of the various types of carbohydrates, proteins, and lipids.

breads, pastas, starches, cakes, cookies, candies, and other industrialized products), as well as containing refined vegetable oils (easily susceptible to oxidation), artificially hydrogenated vegetable fats (containing harmful trans fats), processed meats containing preserving chemicals, and other refined foods deprived of important vitanutrients. Most of those substances, from a point of view of the long process of human evolution, are novelties to our metabolism, introduced just recently in the human diet along the last century.

Some authors have proposed new forms of food pyramids and also forms involving Greek columns (based on the Mediterranean diet) instead of pyramids. The basic fact is that the information contained in the food guide pyramid is too simplistic, lacking important and fundamental nutritional information details, and it doesn't focus on the important aspects of an optimized nutrition.

The carbohydrates from the various food sources are not equal, as far as body metabolism is concerned, affecting in a different way the blood levels of insulin and glucose, and the hormonal balance of the body. There are many different types of lipids present in foods, and they exert different biochemical functions in body metabolism, some of them being essential for good health. Similarly, the various protein sources supply different amino acid profiles, and they are also accompanied by a diversity of other (good or bad) alimentary substances. It is also of

> Carbohydrates from different food sources affect in a different way the blood levels of insulin and glucose, and the body hormonal balance.

fundamental importance to point out the benefits that the vitamins, minerals, soluble fibers, antioxidant substances, and other vitanutrients provide to our health, when ingested in amounts well above those usually present in foods, including supplements of some natural vitanutrients. Another aspect that deserves special attention is the need to maintain an appropriate body weight, within a healthy range, and the health benefits originating from the regular practice of moderate physical exercise and adequate sleep.

1.6 CALORIC ENERGY EXPENDITURE

*T*he expenditure of calories by the body depends on the momentary level of physical activity. The body reacts to physical activity adjusting its use of energy. Hormones (chemical substances that function as biochemical messengers) such as epinephrine or norepinephrine are released in the blood flow, signaling to the liver and body fatty tissues to liberate the stored energy sources, mainly glucose, fatty acids, and some amino acids, in order to produce work.

> Proteins and lipids from different food sources supply different amino acid profiles and different types of fatty acids, some of which are essential.

In physical terms, one *calorie* (cal) is formally defined as the thermal energy necessary to raise the temperature of one gram (1g) of water by one degree centigrade (1°C), specifically from 14.4°C to 15.5°C (under normal atmospheric pressure). In nutrition, however, the term *alimentary calorie* is usually used to represent a thousand physical calories, that is, one alimentary calorie is equivalent to 1,000cal or 1kcal. To have a general notion, one alimentary calorie (1kcal) corresponds approximately to the energy consumed by a medium person (about 75kg of weight) during one minute, under rest conditions (basal metabolism). Therefore, in nutritional terms, a medium person at rest (sleeping) spends about 60 alimentary calories per hour (or 1,440kcal/day).

> One alimentary calorie corresponds approximately to the energy expended, during one minute, by an average person at rest.

Table 1.1 shows average levels of caloric energy used by the body, during one hour, when performing different tasks or physical exercises, typical of a person with a body weight around 75kg. More, or less, body weight, correspondingly will also be your calorie consumption for each physical activity.

TABLE 1.1 – Average calorie expenditure for various physical activities performed during one hour by a medium person with a typical body weight of about 75kg.

ACTIVITY	CALORIES	ACTIVITY	CALORIES
Baseball	300	Piano playing	150
Basketball	450	Ping-pong	270
Bowling	260	Raquetball	600
Canoeing	600	Running (10km/h)	800
Carpentry	400	Scrubbing floors	200
Cycling (8km/h)	170	Sitting (watching TV)	90
Cycling (15km/h)	350	Skiing (snow)	650
Dancing (moderately)	340	Skiing (water)	500
Dancing (vigorously)	400	Sleeping (basal metabolism)	60
Desk work	110	Standing	110
Driving a car	170	Swimming (leisurely)	360
Driving a motorcycle	200	Swimming (competition)	650
Football	600	Tennis	420
Gardening moderately	220	Volleyball	350
Golf	300	Walking (3km/h)	180
Horseback riding	450	Walking (5km/h)	250

To have an approximate idea of the daily expenditure of calories by an adult person, Table 1.2 shows ranges of calorie expenditure, as a function of body weight, representative of persons with small muscular mass and low physical activity levels (column A), persons with medium muscular mass and medium physical activity levels (column B), and persons with large muscular mass and high physical activity levels (column C). Although the

> Our daily calorie expenditure depends on physical activity levels, body weight, and on hormonal and genetic factors.

presented ranges are relatively wide, they provide an adequate indication of daily calorie expenditure, for reference. On the other hand, it is possible to calculate your daily calorie expenditure multiplying the time (in hours) expended in each of your daily activities by the corresponding calorie expenditure of each activity (presented in Table 1.1) and adding the results.

TABLE 1.2 – Ranges of typical average values representative of expended calories per day as a function of body weight, muscular mass, and physical activity levels, for men and women.

MEN			
WEIGHT (kg)	**A**	**B**	**C**
50	1,500 – 1,800	1,700 – 2,200	1,900 – 2,500
60	1,600 – 1,900	1,800 – 2,400	2,000 – 2,700
70	1,700 – 2,000	1,900 – 2,600	2,200 – 3,000
80	1,800 – 2,200	2,100 – 2,800	2,400 – 3,200
90	1,900 – 2,400	2,200 – 2,900	2,500 – 3,400
100	2,000 – 2,500	2,300 – 3,000	2,600 – 3,500

WOMEN			
WEIGHT (kg)	**A**	**B**	**C**
40	1,200 – 1,500	1,400 – 1,700	1,500 – 1,900
50	1,300 – 1,600	1,500 – 1,800	1,600 – 2,000
60	1,400 – 1,700	1,600 – 1,900	1,700 – 2,100
70	1,500 – 1,800	1,700 – 2,000	1,800 – 2,300
80	1,600 – 1,900	1,800 – 2,100	1,900 – 2,400

Note: Column A refers to persons with small muscular mass and low physical activity levels; Column B refers to persons with medium muscular mass and medium physical activity levels; and Column C to persons with large muscular mass and very active physically.

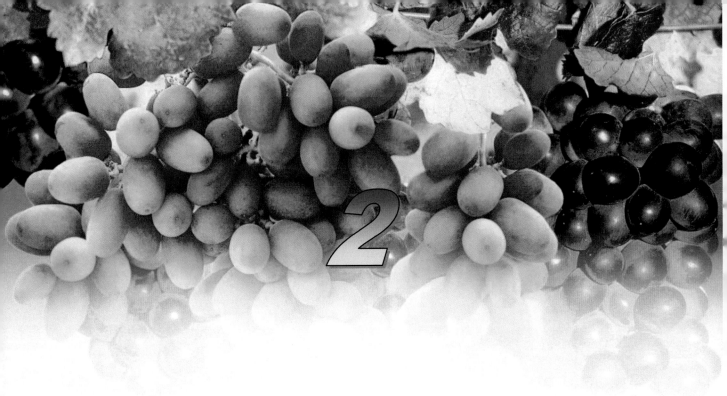

NUTRITION GUIDELINES

2.1 GENERAL PRINCIPLES FOR AN OPTIMUM DIET

Current evidence suggests that, for the maintenance of good health and an appropriate body weight, the best alimentary (nourishment) diet is one that contains approximately 30% of proteins, 30% of lipids, and 40% of carbohydrates (proportions relative to the total of ingested calories), together with the necessary and optimum amounts of vitamins, minerals, soluble fibers, essential fatty acids, and antioxidant substances. For example, for a 2,000 (alimentary) calorie diet, these amounts would be 150g of proteins (that supply about 4 calories/g), 66g of lipids (9 calories/g), and 200g of carbohydrates (4 calories/g). However, some people may not be able to adapt to this macronutrient combination. In this case, they should seek a program that is better for their biotype and genetic predisposition, either by experimenting or based on updated nutritional orientation.

Besides these relative proportions, it is of fundamental importance to observe the quality of the ingested foods. In other words, choose: (1) unrefined whole carbohydrates that have a low *glycemic index* (that is, a low rate of glucose absorption in the bloodstream); (2) complete proteins that contain all the *essential amino acids* in adequate amounts; and (3) unrefined and stable lipids, not susceptible to oxidation, that contain the *essential fatty acids*, being important to avoid fried foods (delicate oils heated to high temperatures for long periods) and artificially *hydrogenated vegetable fats*. For most people, this macronutrient combination allows a healthy maintenance of body tissues and healthy levels of glucose and insulin in the bloodstream, and also of *prostaglandins*, one of the most powerful and important hormonal systems (of short reach and duration) of the human body. The total of ingested calories should be in balance with the total of calories expended daily by the body (or slightly less, in case you need to lose weight). The total number of calories expended daily by the body depends on physical activity levels and on some hormonal and genetic factors.

> Current evidence suggests a daily diet that contains approximately 30% of proteins, 30% of lipids, and 40% of carbohydrates, in terms of ingested calories.

Other factors may also influence the individual need for nutrients. The stress caused by the environment (exposure to atmosphere pollution and some food toxins) and the physical-emotional stress (lifestyle) increase the need of proteins and essential fatty acids, as well as of antioxidant and protecting vitanutrients, such as vitamins C and E, complex B vitamins, beta-carotene, and minerals (as magnesium, zinc, chromium, and selenium).

Food digestion and nutrient absorption in the gastrointestinal tract are sensitive to environmental and emotional conditions. To have your meals in conditions of anxiety, nervousness, fatigue, or preoccupation affects the movements of the stomach and can lead to gastrointestinal disturbances. In a person under physical-emotional stress, the digestive secretions are

> It is important to have your meals in conditions of no anxiety or physical-emotional stress, and in a relaxed and calm environment.

reduced, compromising an efficient nutrient absorption. It is important to have your meals in a relaxed and calm environment.

2.2 YOU ARE UNIQUE

Your metabolic rate is as unique as your personality. Each person possesses his/her own genetic predispositions, family traditions, different histories, different alimentary tastes, specific health problems, and different metabolic rates. Therefore, there is no such thing as a common alimentary diet appropriate for everyone. In nutrition, there are general principles, scientifically based, but not rules or laws.

Any alimentary (nourishment) diet should be analyzed observing those principles, but it is necessary to discover what proportion between carbohydrates, proteins, and lipids works best for you. Try to discover the needs dictated by your own biochemistry and lifestyle. If you are able to discover what is unique about your genetic makeup, you will also find out what is unique about you. There seems to be little doubt that we are better adapted for the basic type of diet that our ancestors were submitted for many hundreds of years and that provided longevity to them. Therefore, choose a type of diet (relative need for carbohydrates, proteins, and lipids) that promoted longevity to your ancestors, as well as foods that provide antioxidants, complemented with updated information from nutritional science.

> Try to discover the needs dictated by your own biochemistry and lifestyle, and choose a type of diet that promoted longevity to your ancestors.

2.3 VARIETY AND COLOR

In order to provide a balanced ingestion of the various nutrients needed by the body, it is important to vary the types of foods. No specific food contains the variety of nutrients present in a wide and diverse group of selected foods. In this way, the nutritional deficiencies of certain foods are compensated by some other complementary foods.

It is not advisable to eat the same foods in a routine way, day after day, because it increases the possibility to develop allergies or alimentary intolerances. It is recommended to alternate, along the week, between the various foods available from a large set of foods. Foods that are not organically developed, or that were exposed to the use of pesticides, hormones, or antibiotics during their production (in the case of meat and poultry), may cause body intoxications, when consumed continually for long periods. Some foods may contain pesticide residues, as well as chemical or other added toxins that, when consumed excessively for long periods, can expose our body to toxin levels that are much larger than those considered safe or tolerated by our body's metabolism.

Choose foods that are dense in nutrients, the closest possible to their natural state (organic or minimally processed), and also lacking in pesticides, hormones, and antibiotics. The nutritional density of a given food refers to the amount of proteins, essential fatty acids, vitamins, minerals, phytochemical substances, and antioxidants that it contains, in relation to their calorie content. Nuts and seeds, for instance, in spite of their high-calorie nature, are extremely nutrient dense foods, being rich in many minerals (magnesium, zinc, selenium, and potassium), proteins, complex carbohydrates, alimentary fibers, essential fatty acids, and vitamin E. Fruits and vegetables, particularly those developed organically (without pesticides, fungicides, and herbicides) and in appropriate soils, are also rich in vitamins, minerals, and phytochemical antioxidants, with few calories. Whenever possible, choose lean meats and organic eggs. On the other hand, refined and processed foods are poor in nutrients. Sugars, refined flours, and similar products provide instant calories (mainly from carbohydrates) without any nutritional value, representing empty calories.

Choose foods that are dense in nutrients and the closest possible to their natural state.

Vegetables and fruits, with their variety of colors, are full of phytochemical substances (or vegetable biochemical substances) with antioxidant properties, including pigments called *carotenoids* and *bioflavonoids*, that strengthen our immune system. In general, the more colorful the vegetables and fruits, the higher is the amount of present antioxidants. This is a promising area of nutritional research, and thousands of phytochemical substances have already been identified. The carotenoids, for instance, constitute a group of yellow, orange, and red substances, found in many vegetable foods. The generic name comes from *carrot*, one of the richest foods in this type of substance. The *beta-carotene*, abundant in carrots, is an excellent antioxidant and also one of the safest vitanutrients, as is *lycopene*, present in red tomatoes, for instance. However, the carotenoids are fat-soluble substances and are absorbed efficiently by the body only when eaten together with foods that contain fats.

Other relevant carotenoids are *lutein* and *zeaxanthin* (of yellowish coloration) that protect our eyes from countless of aggressive agents. They are found in leafy vegetables of dark-green color, as spinach and collard greens, and in egg yolks.

> Vegetables and fruits, with their variety of colors, are full of antioxidant phytochemical substances.

Many herbs and spices, used normally to give flavor to foods, are important sources of minerals and pigments containing bioflavonoids. In general, fresh or frozen foods present larger amounts of antioxidants than canned and processed foods, or foods heated to high temperatures. Also, raw or microwave (slowly) cooked foods are better than the ones cooked in boiling water. Whole fruits are better than fruit juices. It is also important to wash fruits and vegetables appropriately in order to remove any possible chemical or pesticide residue present on their skin.

2.4 DIETARY SUPPLEMENTS

*T*here are many factors that contribute to diminish the nutritional content of foods. The nutritional content of foods depends on the nature of the soil where they were grown. A soil poor in nutrients results in foods also poor in nutrients. Many important substances are removed from the soil by excessive cultivation, acid rain, and indiscriminate use of inorganic fertilizers, agricultural defensives, and pesticides. Exhausted soils reduce the nutritional value of vegetables, in general, and the existing pesticides may provoke the appearance of neurodegenerative diseases and cancer. Industrial processing and refinement also leads to a decrease in the nutritional value of foods, as well as the cooking process. Canned foods are usually deficient in nutrients. Essentially, the modern dietary habits turn common the nutritional deficiencies in the body. In addition, modern lifestyle (pollutants present in the atmosphere and in food, high stress levels, presence of electronic and magnetic radiations, smoke of cigarettes, use of antibiotics, excess alcohol consumption, and use of medicines that block the action of nutrients in the body) increases the need of nutrients well beyond the minimum recommendations normally established to avoid diseases.

Countless studies have confirmed that supplements of vitamins, minerals, and antioxidants can be beneficial, in general, even allied to a selective and optimized natural diet. Although the understanding and recognition of the importance of a selective diet is increasing, many people still don't eat balanced meals in a consistent way. Older people are particularly vulnerable, since, with age, the body gradually loses its ability to digest and absorb nutrients. Research has demonstrated that, most of the time, besides a good selective diet, supplementation may be essential to prevent and treat diseases, in a general way, and to extend life.

Many people believe that the nutrients must be supplied exclusively through a natural diet and that the dietary supplements simply generate a nutrient-rich and expensive urine. The fact that the excess of some nutrients are not stored in the body does not mean that they don't exert important biochemical body functions, but, mainly, that they must be ingested continually to maintain the tissues replenished. You certainly will not stop drinking water, for instance, simply because the body eliminates it through the urine. The nutrients circulate throughout the body, participating in enzyme activation, helping metabolism, neutralizing free radicals (thus, protecting cells and tissues from oxidation), and avoiding the appearance of possible degenerative diseases. A nutrient-rich urine is a good sign, indicating that the body is well supplied with nutrients, as well as protecting important organs such as the bladder and kidneys.

The nutritional content of foods depends on the nature of the soil where they were grown.

Furthermore, practically all comparative studies have demonstrated that people who take supplements are healthier and live longer than those that don't. The supplements of vitamins, minerals, antioxidants, amino acids, and so on, don't produce results immediately. The regeneration or modification in body biochemistry, necessary to repair the nutritional deficiencies, do not occur in a short period, and it may take weeks or months in order to notice the improvements and benefits of an optimized nutrition.

Vitamin supplements may be synthetic or from natural sources. At molecular levels in the body, both forms are equally effective, with a few exceptions, such as vitamin E that should, preferably, be from natural sources for a more efficient absorption. The vitamins A, D, E, and K are fat soluble, needing the simultaneous ingestion of foods that contain fats for efficient absorption. However, particularly the vitamins A and D may become toxic if consumed in large doses for long periods. The other vitamins are soluble in water and eventual excessive doses are normally eliminated in the urine, usually not causing intoxication effects. In this case, it is better to consider the use of timed-release supplements or use smaller doses distributed along the day. It is always advisable, when consuming vitamin and mineral supplements, to have the orientation of a nutritionist or health professional.

> Vitamins A, D, E, and K are fat soluble and need to be ingested simultaneously with foods that contain fat for an efficient absorption.

2.5 LISTENING TO YOUR BODY

It is essential for your health to maintain your body weight within a healthy range. Your weight, relative to your height, as well as your abdominal dimensions, greatly influences your chances to develop high blood pressure, high cholesterol, cardiovascular diseases, diabetes, renal diseases, arthritis, and cancer. Excess weight, besides having a direct negative impact on your present and future health quality, is also a problem that directly influences your personality and self-esteem, and the way people see you and treat you. The fat that accumulates around the waist, or abdominal fat, is usually associated to high blood pressure, high cholesterol, high blood levels of glucose, heart disease, and is also an indicator of eventual health problems later in life. Excess weight, or obesity, refers to excess body fat.

An indication of what is considered a healthy weight is provided by the *Body Mass Index* (BMI). This index is defined as the ratio between your weight (in kilograms) and the square of your height (in meters), that is,

$$BMI = \frac{Weight(kg)}{[Height(m)]^2}$$

For example, a person with 70kg weight and 1.7m tall has a BMI of 24, and a person with 85kg weight and 1.8m tall has a BMI of 26. However, it is also necessary to consider that some people may have more weight due to more athletic and developed muscles, and not due to excess body fat. In terms of caloric balance, the goal should be to reach the weight range adequate to your physical type, and to adopt an alimentary diet and physical activity level that maintain your weight within the healthy range.

The determination of the healthy range of BMIs has been made through the analysis of the mortality rates in large groups of people and selecting the range of BMIs with the smaller mortality rates. This process leads to a U-shaped curve, in which the mortality rates increase in both directions starting from a minimum. Countless studies, that include more than a million adults, show that BMIs above 25 increase the risk of dying prematurely, mainly from heart disease and cancer. There is a consensus that people with a BMI between 25 and 30 are considered above the healthy weight range and above 30 are obese. Weights considered healthy are those associated with BMIs between approximately 19 and 25, with an average around 22. However, the lower part of the curve (BMIs below 19) requires careful analysis. Some specialists state that the curves indicate exactly what they show, that is, a low weight relative to your height also increases the chances of dying prematurely. Other specialists argue that many people are skinny as a result of diseases that lead to weight loss, and people that smoke cigarettes tend to be thinner due to lack of appetite, and smoking represents a great risk of dying prematurely. Therefore, in a large population of skinny people there may be a mixture of healthy skinny people and those that are skinny due to diseases. In other words, BMIs below 19 in healthy people do not necessarily indicate a risk of dying prematurely, and a closer analysis is necessary.

The bottom line is, if your BMI is between 19 and 25, try to maintain it in that *healthy range*, preferably around 22 (see Table 2.1 and Figure 2.1). If it is above 25, consider reducing it to the healthy range.

TABLE 2.1 – Typical values (in kg) for minimum healthy weight (BMI = 19), ideal weight (BMI = 22), and maximum healthy weight (BMI = 25), as a function of height (in meters).

HEIGHT	MINIMUM	IDEAL	MAXIMUM	HEIGHT	MINIMUM	IDEAL	MAXIMUM
1.56	46	54	61	1.74	58	67	76
1.58	47	55	62	1.76	59	68	77
1.60	49	56	64	1.78	60	70	79
1.62	50	58	66	1.80	62	71	81
1.64	51	59	67	1.82	63	73	83
1.66	52	61	69	1.84	64	75	85
1.68	54	62	71	1.86	66	76	87
1.70	55	64	72	1.88	67	78	88
1.72	56	65	74	1.90	69	79	90

In order to lose weight (to burn part of the fat stored in the body) it is essential to limit the ingested calories to a level less (but not much) than the total of expended calories. Select foods that are rich in nutrients and relatively low in calories (with a high nutrient/calorie ratio), and that leads to healthy levels of blood glucose and insulin. The following chapters detail the biochemical properties of the nutrients present in food (particularly the different types of carbohydrates, proteins, and

> Try to maintain your BMI in the healthy range, between 19 and 25, preferably around 22.

It is advisable to maintain a count of the total of daily ingested calories, in order to keep this total slightly below the daily expended calories. This will allow you to develop a practical notion of the relative caloric value of portions of some foods. It is important also to have a reasonable notion of the relative content of carbohydrates, proteins, and fats of the most usual foods, so that you may select foods in a balanced way.

Physical exercise increases the amount of expended calories while burning body fat and developing lean muscular mass. Without exercise, body fat gradually replaces your muscular mass. When exercising, be aware of your physical limitations and do not exceed your natural limits. Avoid excess of stressing aerobic exercise that increases the production of free radicals in the body. Nevertheless, as shown in the next chapters, there are other factors that influence your caloric expenditure and rate of body fat burning, such as genetic factors, hormonal balance, and life style.

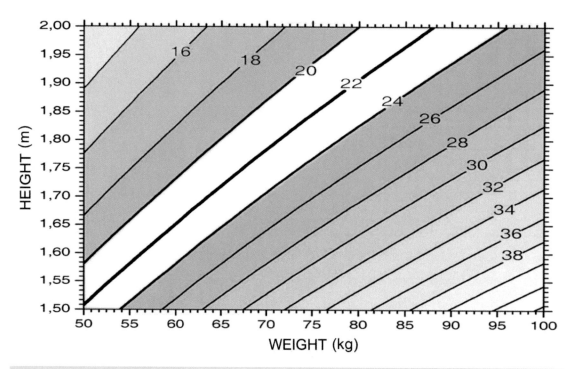

FIGURE 2.1 – Curves of Body Mass Index (BMI) as a function of height (in meters) and body weight (in kg).

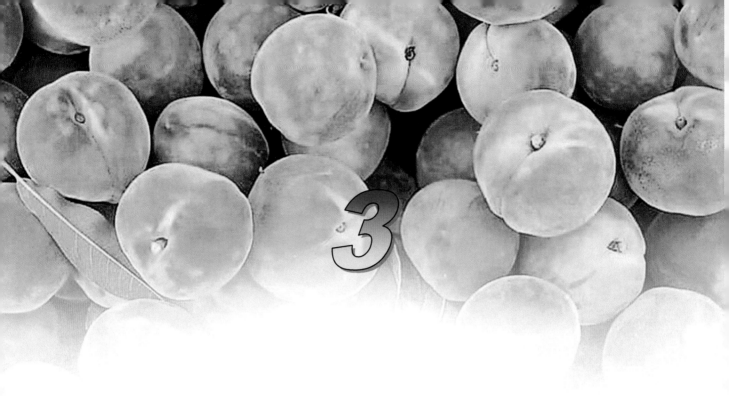

3

CARBOHYDRATES

3.1 ENERGY SOURCES FOR THE BODY

Carbohydrates are foods rich in sugars or sugar complexes (starches) that are used by the body as energy sources for all its functions. They are also called *carbon hydrates* or *glycosides*. Their energy potential is expressed in *calories*, a unit that measures the amount of chemical energy released as heat during food metabolism. Approximately four calories per gram are released during oxidation or combustion of elementary carbohydrates in the interior of cells.

The way that the sugar molecules are grouped together is what determines if a food is classified as a *simple* or a *complex* carbohydrate. These substances are constituted of the chemical elements carbon (C), hydrogen (H), and oxygen (O), and present chemical formulas represented generically by $C_n(H_2O)_m$ (where *n* and *m* denote integer numbers, equal to or greater than 3), that is, apparently, hydrate of carbon. For example, the single sugars *glucose*, *fructose*, and *galactose* possess the chemical formula $C_6H_{12}O_6$ and *sucrose*

$C_{12}H_{22}O_{11}$. Regardless of their name, there are no water (H_2O) molecules in carbohydrates, but the carbon atoms are attached to each other (as a chain) and to atoms of hydrogen, oxygen, and the *hydroxyl* group or radical –OH. In organic chemistry, the term *radical* refers to a molecular fragment. The denomination carbon hydrate was originally introduced by the French (*hydrate de carbone*) that, although inadequate, continued to be used in the form carbohydrate.

> Carbohydrates are composed of sugars and sugar polymers, and they provide about four calories per gram in the metabolic burning process.

For illustration purposes, the chemical formula of *glucose* is presented in Figure 3.1, in which the carbon and (one) oxygen atoms form a six-sided (hexagonal) ring. In this representation, the lines between atoms indicate *chemical bonds*, so that a single line represents a single bond. Carbon binds chemically through four bonds (valence 4), oxygen through two bonds (valence 2), and hydrogen through one bond (valence 1). Glucose is the most abundant simple carbohydrate in nature and supplies energy to cells in the body. It is also referred to as *dextrose*.

3.2 SUGARS AND STARCHES

The main substances that constitute the carbohydrates are *sugars* and *starches*. They are systematically classified as *monosaccharides*, *disaccharides*, and *polysaccharides*. The word *saccharide* is derived from Greek (*sakkharon*) and means "sugar". Sugars are divided into two categories: monosaccharides, which are single sugars composed of one molecule; and disaccharides, which are composed of two monosaccharide molecules chemically joined by a process called *condensation* (a process in which a covalent bond is formed between two molecules by removal of a water molecule). Starches are complex carbohydrates, composed of many different combinations of chains (polymers) of monosaccharides interconnected through glycosidic bonds, and are denominated

> Starches are polysaccharides composed of polymeric chains of monosaccharides (single sugars).

polysaccharides. Glucose is the basic unit of polysaccharides. The term *oligosaccharide* is used to indicate a small polymer that contains some groups of interconnected monosaccharides.

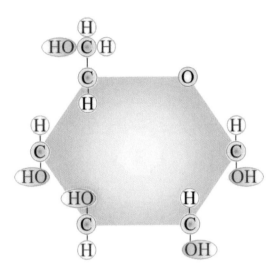

FIGURE 3.1 – The chemical formula of glucose forms a six-sided (hexagonal) ring.

Most of natural monosaccharides contain five or six carbon atoms in their molecular chain and are denominated *pentoses* or *hexoses*, respectively. The most common monosaccharides in the human diet and of nutritional interest are: (1) *glucose* (also known as blood sugar); (2) *fructose* (found mainly in fruits); and (3) *galactose* (liberated during digestion of milk). Our liver metabolism can convert fructose and galactose into glucose. They all are hexoses and have the same chemical formula $C_6H_{12}O_6$, but each has a different spatial arrangement of atoms. The spatial structure of galactose is similar to that of glucose, except that the hydroxyl group of the fourth carbon atom, counted clockwise from the oxygen atom in the ring, is spatially oriented in opposition to that of glucose (see Figure 3.2). In food, galactose usually occurs in a disaccharide molecule, bonded to glucose to form lactose (the

> Glucose, fructose, and galactose have the same chemical formula, but have different spatial structures and biochemical properties.

primary sugar in milk). Fructose tastes the sweetest of all the sugars and is naturally present in honey, some vegetables, and many fruits. It is also called *levulose* or fruit sugar. The spatial chemical structure of fructose is somewhat different from that of glucose and galactose, as it consists of a five-sided (pentagon) ring (see Figure 3.3).

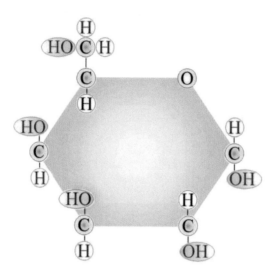

FIGURE 3.2 – The chemical formula of galactose is similar to that of glucose, except for the different spatial orientation of one of the –OH radicals (compare to Figure 3.1).

The many different possible spatial orientations of the groups of atoms in the monosaccharide molecules give rise to spatial isomers or *stereoisomers* that have different biochemical properties. Glucose, fructose, and galactose are, therefore, natural spatial *isomers*, or *stereoisomers*, that is, they have the same chemical formula, but differ in their spatial structure and also in their biochemical properties. The monosaccharides that have chemical formulas with a six-sided (hexagonal) ring, for example, constitute 16 stereoisomers, divided

The many different possible spatial orientations of the groups of atoms in the monosaccharide molecules give rise to stereoisomers.

into two groups of eight (denominated *glucose, galactose, mannose, allose, altrose, gulose, idose*, and *talose*), which may occur as D (*dextro*-rotation) or L (*levo*-rotation) optical isomers (mirror images, such as the right and left hands). A relevant fact is that most of the hexoses present in living organisms are in the isomeric form D. Our body, for instance, can only use the D-isomer of saccharides.

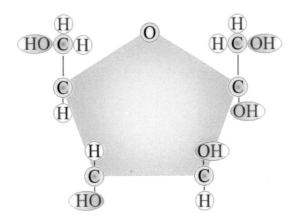

FIGURE 3.3 – The chemical formula of fructose forms a five-sided (pentagon) ring.

Pentoses (single sugar molecules that contain five carbon atoms) are present in foods in only small quantities, but they are essential components of nucleic acids, which are the genetic material of life (as *ribose* and *deoxyribose*).

The disaccharides of nutritional interest are: (1) *sucrose* (common table sugar, purified from sugar cane or beets), which is broken, during digestion, into the monosaccharides glucose and fructose (2) *lactose* (milk sugar), which is broken, during digestion, into the monosaccharides glucose and galactose; and (3) *maltose* (a breakdown product of starches and cereals), which is a glucose-glucose disaccharide. The breakdown of disaccharides into monosaccharides is done by the *hydrolysis* process, adding a water molecule (H_2O) in the process.

Honey is basically constituted of sucrose, with traces of some vitamins and minerals.

Starches are constituted of two types of glucose polymers, called *amylose* and *amylopectin*. Amylose is a linear polymer formed of non-ramified long chains of chemically-joined D-glucose molecules, whereas amylopectin is also formed with long D-glucose chains, but the chains are highly ramified. Examples include cereals, legumes, and tubers (such as rice, beans, soy, wheat, grains, potatoes, and manioc). During digestion, starches are broken by the saliva and gastric juice enzymes, through hydrolysis, finally liberating the single sugar molecules. Some natural complex carbohydrates (unrefined) require, in general, a longer digestion time for the enzymes to break down the polysaccharides into single sugar molecules and, finally, into glucose for absorption.

Fibers are present in many natural (unrefined) complex carbohydrates and they may be soluble in water or insoluble. They are constituted of polysaccharides such as cellulose (e.g., cotton and paper), resins, pectins, and mucilages, and are practically not digested and do not provide energy. Nevertheless, the alimentary fibers play an important role in the health of the gastrointestinal tract.

In general, the simple carbohydrates (like sugar, honey, and maltose), as well as some refined carbohydrates or starches (like white rice, white flour and derivatives, potatoes, and manioc) are easily digested and their glucose is rapidly absorbed into the bloodstream after ingestion, causing rapid fluctuations in the glucose blood levels. On the other hand, some complex carbohydrates (such as beans, soy, peas, peanuts, nuts, seeds, and integral grains) require a much longer time in order to be digested and their glucose enters the bloodstream in a slow and gradual way, therefore, not causing abrupt changes in the blood levels of glucose and in the body energy flow. This is one of the major reasons why unrefined complex carbohydrates are considered much healthier than simple ones, besides being rich in alimentary fibers and possibly containing some vitamins and

> The simple and refined carbohydrates are easily digested and their glucose enters rapidly in the bloodstream after ingestion.

minerals. The refined complex carbohydrates (such as white rice, white flour, and products that contain it) are considered low quality from a nutritional point of view, since they were deprived of important vitanutrients and alimentary fibers, remaining only polysaccharides that our body quickly converts into glucose.

The single sugars, resulting from the chemical decomposition of carbohydrates in the gastrointestinal tract, are absorbed in the bloodstream through capillaries in the intestinal walls. Most of it goes to the *portal vein*, the great

> The glucose molecules are oxidized inside the cell mitochondria, which are tiny power plants for energy production.

blood vessel that conducts the nutrients to the liver. The liver receives and transforms the single sugars into glucose. In the bloodstream, the glucose is transported to all body cells, where it is oxidized (burned) inside the *mitochondria* (small structures inside the cells that act as power plants for energy production), through a complex cycle of metabolic reactions, providing the necessary energy for muscles, tissues, brain, nervous system, biochemical processes, and to maintain a warm body temperature. This cellular combustion process, besides energy, also produces water (H_2O) and carbon dioxide (CO_2) that are transported in the bloodstream and eliminated by the kidneys, lungs, and sweat. The liver also produces glucose from the lactic acid liberated from the glucose burning process, when the muscles work with low levels of oxygen.

3.3 THE INSULIN HORMONE

*T*he *insulin* hormone is produced by the pancreas to process the glucose in the blood, controlling its use, distribution, and energy storage in the body. When the blood glucose level rises, as a result of the ingestion of carbohydrates, a group of endocrine cells in the pancreas (known as *islets of Langerhans*) secrete insulin to process and transport glucose to the various body cells. The word insulin derives from *insula*, or *island*, a name originating from the islets that contain

> Insulin processes glucose in the blood, controlling its use, distribution, and energy storage.

the cells secreting insulin and that are surrounded by tissues.

An amount of glucose that is not immediately necessary for energy production is transformed into *glycogen*, which is temporally stored in the muscles, liver, and in smaller quantities in all cells, until the body demands its mobilization. Glycogen is a type of animal starch, that is, a storage polysaccharide in animal cells. The stored glycogen represents a reserve that our body can use in case of need between meals and during sleep. This reserve contains about 2,000 calories, which is enough for about two days. Residues of fats, proteins, and other substances taken to the liver are also used to produce the glycogen macromolecules.

> The glycogen stored in the tissues constitutes a polysaccharide reserve that contains about 2,000 calories.

The remaining glucose in the blood is reprocessed in the liver and can be converted into small fat particles called *triglycerides*, which constitute the raw material for the fat stored in the body. Our body can synthesize fats starting from carbohydrates, through a complex enzymatic metabolic process involving the production of an intermediate substance called *acetyl-coenzyme A* (or *acetyl-coA*). This synthesis occurs mainly in the liver and in the cellular cytoplasm, when the cells have abundance of energy. Acetyl-coA is also the raw material for the synthesis of cholesterol.

The triglycerides are small and light fat particles constituted of three molecules of fatty acids joined to a glycerol backbone (see the chapter on lipids). Part of the triglycerides are incorporated into blood *lipoproteins* (see the chapter on cholesterol and lipoproteins) known as *Very-Low Density Lipoproteins* (VLDL). Together with other blood lipids, these substances are considered potentially harmful when present in excess in the blood, especially when oxidized. Triglyceride blood levels are usually used as prognosticators of the risk of developing cardiovascular diseases. Excess fat stored mainly in the waist region (intra-abdominal fat) and high blood levels of triglycerides

> Starting from carbohydrates, our body can synthesize triglycerides, which constitute the raw material for the fat stored in the body.

represent a large risk of cardiovascular problems.

The blood levels of glucose and insulin vary according to the type of ingested carbohydrate. One of the important functions of the adrenal glands is to regulate the blood glucose level. Our body tends to maintain this level within a relatively small range, normally between 65mg and 110mg of glucose per cubic centimeter of blood. It is at those levels that the body is adapted and functions better as a result of hundreds of thousands of years of evolution. During the extremely slow human evolution process, the human body was molded and adapted through the ingestion of natural unrefined carbohydrates, besides fats and proteins of both animal and vegetal origin.

Our body is simply not adapted for the exaggerated consumption of sugars and refined carbohydrates (products that contain white flour) that has occurred over the last century and still today. After the ingestion of foods rich in sugars and refined carbohydrates, excess glucose rapidly enters the bloodstream and the body secretes large quantities of insulin to process all this glucose. This causes large variations in the blood

> Our body tries to maintain the glucose level in the blood within a relatively narrow range, about 65mg to 110mg per cm^3 of blood.

levels of glucose and insulin, during each ingestion, causing excess glucose to be converted into triglycerides. High blood triglyceride levels contribute to body fat, obesity, and cardiovascular diseases. Proteins have little effect in the insulin and glucose blood levels, whereas the alimentary fats have practically no effect.

3.4 HYPERINSULINISM AND INSULIN RESISTANCE

A high blood insulin level is one of the factors that promote obesity and heart disease, and chronic situations can lead to diabetes. When we ingest large quantities of carbohydrates (refined or whole ones) there will be a lot of glucose available to the body and the excess glucose (not necessary for momentarily energy or glycogen generation) will be converted into fat (including triglycerides and cholesterol). As more fat is stored in our body, less is the cell's ability to react to insulin. The pancreas secretes insulin to distribute glucose to the cells, but cells do not absorb it. This phenomenon is called *insulin resistance*. The cell resistance to insulin maintains the blood glucose at high levels for longer periods and stimulates extra secretion of insulin to force the glucose to enter the cells. This process gives rise to a *vicious cycle*: with more fat stored in the tissues, larger is the resistance to insulin, which causes extra production of insulin, transformation of excess glucose into fat and increase of the fat stored in the body. The excessive production of insulin can exhaust the pancreas to the point of impairing its normal functioning and leading to diabetes.

> The cell resistance to insulin and glucose absorption leads to extra production of insulin, stressing the pancreas.

Disturbances in the blood levels of insulin and glucose can be damaging to the body. The heart, blood vessels, kidneys, eyes, and nerves are particularly vulnerable. These disturbances may evolve in phases, going from insulin resistance to *diabetes type 2*. People with diabetes type 2 suffer from hyperinsulinism and produce too much insulin, stressing the pancreas. People with *diabetes type 1* have a deficient production of insulin as a result of a damaged pancreas, generally due to genetic defects or other reasons, and need insulin injections. Hyperinsulinism accelerates aging and is one of the main causes of hypertension.

A balanced diet, restricted to moderate amounts of carbohydrates (selecting only the complex and whole varieties, and avoiding sugars and white flour products), can maintain adequate levels of blood insulin and glucose, especially when complemented with minerals such as chromium and zinc, which diminish insulin resistance. Refined carbohydrates such as white flour products,

> Hyperinsulinism accelerates aging, causes hypertension, and may lead to diabetes mellitus.

table sugar, and white rice are deficient in vitamins, minerals, and fiber, and have been denominated as *empty calories*. Excessive ingestion of industrial foods such as sweets, crackers, and white bread can cause nutritional deficiencies (and their undesirable consequences) and promote obesity and hyperinsulinism. These foods may provide immediate energy to the body, as they cause an abrupt increase in the blood glucose level, but when this level decays rapidly (*hypoglycemia*) as a result of excessive insulin production, a hunger is generated for more carbohydrates, together with permanent feelings of fatigue, nervousness, irritability, and headaches.

3.5 CONSEQUENCES OF CARBOHYDRATE EXCESS

Complex, unrefined carbohydrates, in their natural form, present many health benefits, because they provide energy, contain alimentary fibers, and may be good sources of vitamins and minerals (depending on the soil where they were grown). The same does not apply to the refined carbohydrates and simple sugars. However, even the complex, unrefined carbohydrates are beneficial only in limited amounts, adequate to each organism. Each person has a proper individual need for carbohydrates.

> Excessive intake of carbohydrates may result in a variety of health problems.

Sedentary people need fewer carbohydrates than those that practice physical exercise regularly. Also, our need for carbohydrates diminishes as we get older.

To overload the body with carbohydrates may result in a number of health problems:

➤ Production of excessive blood levels of insulin (hyperinsulinism), triglycerides, and cholesterol, causing gain in body fat, swelling, hunger for more carbohydrates, headaches, and permanent fatigue.
➤ Promotion of obesity, cardiovascular diseases, and diabetes.
➤ Damaging of tissue proteins, through the glycation process, causing precocious cellular aging.
➤ Increase of the need for complex B vitamins, zinc, and chromium.
➤ Weakening of blood capillary vessels.
➤ Stressing the adrenal glands (that regulates the blood glucose level) to an exhaustion state, thus compromising the blood glucose balance.

➢ Together with low-fat diets, not providing adequate amounts of essential fatty acids, compromising the normal functioning of the brain and nervous system, and the balance of the system of prostaglandins (essential for good health).

➢ Together with low-fat diets, causing damage to the liver.

➢ Displacing protein absorption necessary for tissue formation and repair, energy production, immunological functions, and maintenance of blood glucose balance.

Excessive ingestion of refined carbohydrates and simple sugars leaves the body vulnerable to weaknesses and diseases, causing the suppression of the immune system in many ways:

➢ Diminishing the production of antibodies in the bloodstream.

➢ Destroying the capacity of the white blood cells to kill invading germs, for up to five hours after ingestion.

➢ Interfering with the transport of vitamin C in the body, one of the most important vitanutrients and antioxidants.

➢ Causing an unbalance of minerals and, sometimes, allergic reactions.

➢ Making cells more permeable and, consequently, more vulnerable to invading microorganisms, through the neutralization of the action of essential fatty acids.

➢ Increasing the levels of free radicals and creating an environment for the development of pathogenic elements and infections by fungi (such as *Candida Albicans*, for example).

If you ingest more calories than the body expends, you will gain body fat. However, to drastically restrict calorie intake may lead to many undesirable consequences. In a situation of caloric privation, in which the total calorie ingested is much lower than what our body needs, the body may reduce its metabolism and the potential for fat burning (recognizing a situation of extreme food shortage), and may even store body fat to guarantee self preservation and subsistence in the long term, with generalized health damage.

3.6 SUGAR: WHEN SWEET BECOMES BITTER

Sugar (sucrose or table sugar) represents the number one antinutrient and can cause a series of harmful consequences to our health. Some nutritionists affirm that to ingest sugar is somewhat analogous to hit your own head. When consumed sporadically and in small quantities, by healthy people, the body recovers, but exaggerations can be harmful.

As well-documented in the literature, sugar has the property to increase the blood levels of insulin, triglycerides, and cholesterol, and the tendency of blood to coagulate. It promotes the blockage of arteries, suppresses the immune system, and exhausts the adrenal glands (that balances blood sugar levels) and the pancreas (that secretes insulin). Even more, it inhibits the absorption of the B-complex vitamins and the minerals chromium and zinc, interferes in the absorption of calcium and magnesium, increases blood pressure, increases the risk for breast cancer, damages the kidneys, promotes arthritis, causes headaches and migraines, increases stomach acidity, contributes to obesity, provokes fatigue and cravings for more sugar, and favors the growth of fungi and candida.

High blood levels of triglycerides and cholesterol increase the risk for cardiovascular diseases. High insulin levels increase the tendency of cholesterol to adhere to the blood vessel walls. Sugar helps saturated fats contribute for the increase of blood cholesterol levels. It also decreases the amount of bacteria that help to maintain normal cholesterol levels and harms the immune system. Sugar interferes, in a prejudicial way, in the antioxidant activity of the vitamins C and E, which protect against the oxidation of cholesterol by free radicals. Countless evidences demonstrate the connection between sugar consumption and the increase in cardiovascular diseases. It is also known that cancerous cells consume sugar.

> Sugar represents the number one antinutrient and can cause a variety of harmful consequences to our health.

Sucrose (table sugar or honey) is a disaccharide and its body metabolism generates in the first step (hydrolysis process) equal quantities of glucose and fructose ($C_{12}H_{22}O_{11} + H_2O \longrightarrow C_6H_{12}O_6 + C_6H_{12}O_6$). The glucose goes directly to the metabolic processes that provide energy to the body cells, through insulin. The fructose metabolism, however, follows a different path, participating in the formation of an intermediate substance, which is a precursor for cholesterol synthesis by the liver. The excess glucose in the blood and cells may also contribute to the synthesis of triglycerides and cholesterol. Many clinical studies have clearly shown that the ingestion of sucrose leads to an increase in the blood cholesterol levels. It is well known that the correlation between cardiovascular disease and sugar intake is much more significant than that related to excess fat intake.

There seems to be little doubt that the large increase in sucrose consumption that has occurred during the last century, to which our body was not previously adapted, is the cause of many diseases. The increase in the incidence of coronary disease in modern times is somewhat linked to the increase in sucrose consumption (as well as of refined carbohydrate consumption) and it does not seem to be related to animal fat or total fat consumption. A large scale and long duration study performed in the population of Framingham, Massachusetts, conducted by the National Health Institute, starting in 1970, showed no correlation between the ingestion of saturated (animal) fat and the incidence of cardiovascular disease in healthy people.

A reduction in the ingestion of sucrose can improve our health and diminish the risk of developing cardiovascular diseases, diabetes, and other diseases, lowering the blood levels of triglycerides and cholesterol, and strengthening the body natural defense mechanisms (immune system). Some good habits for sucrose ingestion reduction include: (1) stay away from table sugar; (2) do not eat sugary cereals as those industrially made for breakfast (such as corn or rice flake cereals); (3) do not eat sweets/desserts regularly; and (4) do not consume soft

> Sugar, in its various forms, should be avoided and consumed minimally on special occasions.

drinks or fruit juices with added sugar. Essentially, sugar should be avoided at all costs and consumed minimally on special occasions.

Similarly, artificial sweeteners should be used minimally because their effects on the body over a long period are unknown and their consumption reinforces the need for a sweet flavor. If you crave to eat sweets, choose or make a dessert with low calories, without sugar, and sweetened preferably with *sucralose* or *stevia* sweeteners. Sucralose is artificially made from sucrose. It is non-nutritive and hundreds of times sweeter than sugar. Stevia is a natural sweetener, also called stevioside, extracted from the leaves of the Stevia plant. It is also much sweeter than sugar and is not metabolized by the body.

> In case you choose to use artificial sweeteners, give preference to sweeteners based on sucralose or stevia.

Although the natural (unrefined) sugars such as honey, brown sugar, and rice or corn syrups may demand less from the adrenal glands than white sugar (sucrose), they are almost as bad as the latter, causing all the harms already mentioned. Also, concentrated fruit juices are rich in fructose and they don't provide the benefits of the whole fruit itself. On the other hand, vegetables and fruits that contain small amounts of sugar supply vitamins, minerals, valuable phenolic compounds, antioxidants, essential fatty acids, and soluble fibers, and contribute to promote good health when consumed as part of a balanced diet. Milk contains high amounts of lactose (a glucose-galactose disaccharide) and should be consumed with moderation, besides the fact that many people do not appropriately digest lactose or are allergic to milk. A lot of people do not produce the *lactase* enzyme necessary for lactose metabolism. Cheeses and yogurts (fermented milk derivatives) should be consumed as they are excellent sources of complete proteins, vitamins, and minerals (especially calcium), and the processing drastically reduces the amount of lactose in these foods.

> Cheeses and yogurts are excellent sources of complete proteins, vitamins, and minerals, and the fermentation process drastically reduces the amount of lactose in these products.

The bottom line is: be sure to eliminate

all refined junk food from your diet, including table sugar, confectionery, candies, donuts, cookies, cakes, crackers, biscuits, crisps, white bread, French fries, sodas, fruit juices, flavored milks, and all industrial packaged products that contain corn syrup, rice syrup, maple syrup, maltodextrin (glucose polymers), lactose, dextrose (glucose), fructose, maltose, date sugar, cane sugar, corn sugar, and beet sugar.

3.7 IN SUMMARY

Carbohydrate foods are used by the body as energy sources. The main ones are the *sugars* (simple carbohydrates) and the *starches* or sugar polymers (complex carbohydrates). The glucose, from the digestion of these foods, is absorbed in the bloodstream and transported to the many body tissue cells, where it is oxidized (burned) inside the cell *mitochondria*, which are tiny structures inside the cells that act as power plants for energy production.

Glucose processing in the blood is controlled by the *insulin hormone*, secreted by the pancreas. Part of the glucose that is not immediately used for energy is stored as *glycogen* (a type of animal starch) in the body tissues and in the liver, as a short time reserve (equivalent to about 2,000 calories). The remaining glucose is reprocessed in the liver and may be converted into *triglycerides* (a type of fat), which is stored as body fat for eventual posterior use as an energy source, when there is a momentary lack of energy-providing foods.

The more carbohydrates you consume, the more insulin is needed. Excess blood insulin, resulting from excessive intake of easy-absorption carbohydrates, can lead to many severe health problems, including cardiovascular diseases, obesity, and type 2 diabetes mellitus. Obese people develop *cell resistance to insulin*, which requires extra production of insulin by the pancreas to force the glucose into the cells. Besides causing serious damages to the body, the *hyperinsulinism* makes it difficult to lose weight, and it accelerates aging. To increase insulin efficiency, some researchers suggest the consumption of some supplements (such as chromium, zinc, and vitamin E), as well as weight loss.

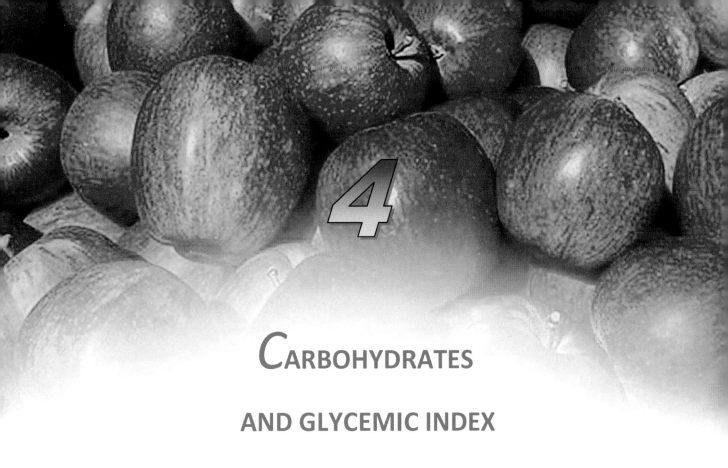

CARBOHYDRATES

AND GLYCEMIC INDEX

4.1 THE GLYCEMIC INDEX

*T*he *glycemic index* (GI) is a relative quantity that indicates the rate (or speed) at which determined carbohydrate food is broken into glucose during digestion and absorbed in the blood. The standard, or reference, to which foods are evaluated, is glucose, which is classified as 100% (some tables may use white bread as reference, classifying it as 100%). This concept applies only to foods rich in carbohydrates. Foods rich in proteins and fats do not cause significant alterations in blood glucose levels.

Foods with a high GI rapidly liberate glucose in the bloodstream. They cause a rapid rise in the blood glucose levels, signaling to the pancreas to secrete extra insulin. These high GI carbohydrate foods must be avoided, as they are fast insulin inductors and cause undesirable fluctuations in the blood levels of glucose and insulin.

Foods with a low GI liberate slowly and gradually the glucose into the bloodstream, providing to the brain and body a more stable and durable energy flow. These low GI carbohydrates are, therefore, much healthier. As a rule, choose carbohydrates with the smaller possible GI. Also, keep in mind that, when proteins, fats, and alimentary fibers are ingested simultaneously with carbohydrate-rich foods, they may cut the rate at which glucose is absorbed into the bloodstream. In fact, one way to ingest high GI carbohydrates and to slow down the glucose absorption is to eat them simultaneously with proteins, fats, and soluble fibers.

> Carbohydrates of high glycemic index quickly liberate glucose in the blood, causing extra production of insulin.

Tables 4.1 and 4.2 present a list of some carbohydrate-rich foods with their corresponding glycemic index, having glucose as reference. Since the metabolism of each person processes foods in slightly different ways, the GI published in tables represent average values. These indices are obtained experimentally through the individual clinical monitoring of a large group of people. Although refined carbohydrates are sometimes listed under the same category as whole grains, the latter are more beneficial, since they were not deprived of vitamins, minerals, and fibers, as a result of industrial refining. Many Internet sites present tables for the GI of carbohydrate-rich foods (search for *glycemic index*).

> As a general rule, choose carbohydrates with the lowest possible glycemic index.

4.2 GLYCEMIC LOAD OF CARBOHYDRATES

*B*esides the glycemic index (GI), it is also important to consider the total amount of carbohydrates present in a determined amount of food (that is, the carbohydrate density). Some authors use the concept of *glycemic load* (GL) obtained multiplying the glycemic index (in percentage) by the amount of carbohydrates present in 100g of that food.

TABLE 4.1 – Glycemic index (GI) of carbohydrate-rich foods and their glycemic load (GL) for 100g of food. Foods with GI below (or equal to) 50.

FOOD	GI	GL	FOOD	GI	GL
Yogurt, plain, no sugar	14	2	Apple juice	40	5
Peanuts	15	4	Fettuccine	40	10
Soybeans	18	2	Chocolate cake	40	20
Fructose	20	20	Wheat germ	41	22
Peas, dry	22	2	Peach	42	5
Cherry	22	3	Pear, canned	43	4
Peanut butter	22	5	Orange	43	5
Cashew nuts	22	6	Lentils, soup	44	4
Chocolate milk, no sugar	24	2	Carrot juice	45	4
Yogurt, lowfat with fruits	24	3	Fermented milk	45	10
Grapefruit	25	3	Capellini	45	11
Barley, grains	25	7	Pinapple juice	46	6
Milk, whole	27	2	Grape	46	7
Beans, kidney	29	7	Linguini	46	12
Plum, dry	29	16	Sponge-cake	46	27
Lentils	30	4	Barley bread	46	30
Beans, black	30	7	Lactose	46	46
Apricot, dry	31	15	Peach, canned	47	4
Milk, lowfat	32	2	Macaroni	47	14
Beans, lima	32	7	Fruit bread	47	23
Yogurt with fruits	33	6	Grapefruit juice	48	5
Chocolate milk with sugar	34	4	Peas, fresh	48	7
Rye, grains	34	26	Grape juice	48	8
Soy milk	36	3	Spaghetti	48	14
Chick-pea	36	8	Bread, mixed grains	48	24
Tomato	38	2	Oatmeal bread	48	25
Tomato juice	38	3	Chocolate bar	49	26
Apple	38	5	Oatmeal	49	36
Pear	38	5	Orange juice	50	5
Plum	39	5	Tortellini with cheese	50	6
Ravioli with meat	39	8	Ice cream, lowfat	50	10
Strawberry	40	3	Pinapple	50	7
Carrot, cooked	40	4	Yam	50	12

TABLE 4.2 – Glycemic index (GI) of carbohydrate-rich foods and their glycemic load (GL) for 100g of food. Foods with GI above 50.

FOOD	GI	GL	FOOD	GI	GL
Banana cake	51	23	Pancake	67	49
Strawberry jelly	51	33	Soft drink with sugar	68	8
Kiwi	53	6	Nhoque	68	18
Banana	54	13	Wheat bread with fiber	68	30
Fruit coquetel	55	8	Table sugar (sucrose)	68	68
Mango	55	8	Wheat cookie	70	54
Whole rice	55	13	Wheat cereal	70	56
Fried potato (industrial)	55	14	Whole wheat bread	71	30
Corn	55	14	Cracker	71	52
Chocolate bar (Snickers)	55	32	Watermelon	72	4
Oatmeal cookie	55	36	Popcorn	72	40
Oatmeal cereal	55	39	Cooked potato	73	18
Musli (cereal)	56	30	Corn cookie	74	42
Apricot	57	5	Cheerios cereal	74	50
Rye bread	58	27	Pumpkin	75	4
Papaya	59	8	French fries	75	19
Pizza (cheese and tomato)	60	16	Waffle	76	29
Ice cream (vanilla)	60	16	Donut	76	36
Honey	60	40	Gatorade	78	5
Sweet potato	61	14	White rice	80	24
Hamburger bread	61	30	Instant oat porridge	80	56
Condensed milk	61	35	Corn cereal	80	70
Muesli bar	61	43	Manioc	81	70
Muffins	62	35	Pretzel	82	63
Beet	64	5	Rice flakes with sugar	82	70
Bean soup	64	7	Corn flakes with sugar	83	70
Apricot, canned	64	10	Roasted potato	85	21
Semolina bread	64	30	Wheat bread, no gluten	85	43
Raisins	64	47	Instant white rice	90	27
Cantaloupe (melon)	65	4	French bread	90	48
Pea soup	66	11	Glucose	100	100
Croissant	67	30	Maltodextrin	105	95
Cake, angel food	67	38	Maltose	105	105

For example, 100g of baked potato (GI of 85% having 25g of carbohydrates) represent a GL of 21, whereas 100g of cooked carrots (GI of 40% with 10g of carbohydrates) represent a GL of 4 and 100g of sugarless yogurt (GI of 14% having 10g of carbohydrates) represent a GL of only 1.4. Values of GL for some carbohydrate-rich foods are also shown in Tables 4.1 and 4.2, considering 100g of food.

Table 4.3 (at the end of this chapter) shows the relative composition of macronutrients of some carbohydrate-rich foods and their calorie content, for reference. On the USDA (US Department of Agriculture) website, there are extensive tables containing the detailed nutritional composition of thousands of foods. The URL is *http://www.ars.usda.gov/ba/bhnrc/ndl*.

4.3 OBESITY AND INSULIN

*O*besity occurs as the result of an abnormal increase in the body fatty tissues. Obese people generally have high blood levels of *insulin*. Since insulin is also involved in the conversion of excess blood glucose into triglycerides and, therefore, in body fat storage, it becomes difficult for obese people to lose weight. Excess insulin increases insulin resistance, making it more difficult for the cells to absorb glucose for energy production. Besides, high insulin levels caused by diets rich in high-GI carbohydrates may block an effective action of the *glucagon* hormone in the body. This peptidic hormone (made of proteins) is essential to make the body fat available for burning.

The glucagon hormone is secreted by the pancreas, and its primary function is to liberate the fat stored in the tissues, allowing the body to burn this fat for energy production. Thus, excess insulin inhibits the glucagon action and denies the body its ability to burn stored fat. On the other hand, proteins stimulate glucagon production by the pancreas. Healthy fats reduce the rate of carbohydrate absorption in the gastrointestinal system, balance prostaglandin

> The glycemic load (GL) refers to the glycemic index (GI) multiplied by the percentage of carbohydrates present in the food.

production (see the chapter on fatty acids and health), and improve the ratio of glucagon to insulin. Diets low in carbohydrates and rich in proteins and healthy fats can restore a healthy balance in the blood levels of insulin and glucose, help to burn the body stored fat, and promote weight loss (as long as the total daily calorie ingestion is adequately limited).

> The peptidic hormone glucagon is fundamental to liberate body fat to be burned for energy production.

According to well-informed nutritionists, obese people should limit their carbohydrate intake to a level well below 40% of the total ingested calories, consuming preferentially low-GI complex carbohydrates. Also, they may benefit from supplements of chromium and zinc (that diminish insulin resistance) and the amino acid *L-carnitine* (that helps the body to burn stored fat). Generally, as less carbohydrate is present in the diet, the better will be for the body to burn body fat. The reduction in carbohydrate ingestion, however, must be gradual and not abrupt, allowing the body to gradually change its hormonal balance.

The amount of fat stored in the body depends directly on the type of ingested food, when they are ingested, and the quantity. Foods of good nutritional quality, spaced in small and more frequent meals, may generate much less body fat as they reduce insulin production. It is important, also, to consume proteins and amino acids (such as L-carnitine) that help to burn body fat and develop lean muscular mass (see the chapter on proteins). An appropriate hormonal balance in the blood levels of insulin, glucagon, and prostaglandins is fundamental to burn body fat. It is not advisable to eat carbohydrates at night, at least for several hours before going to bed, since the body at rest will not need much energy and excess glucose in the body stream will be converted into triglycerides (and body fat).

> To lose weight it is necessary to restrict the total of ingested calories and to avoid the intake of high-GI carbohydrates.

If you ingest more calories than the body expends, you will gain body fat. However, to drastically restrict calorie intake may lead to many undesirable consequences. In a situation of caloric privation, in which the total calorie ingested is much lower than what the body needs, the body may reduce its metabolism and the potential for fat burning (recognizing a situation of extreme food shortage), and may even store body fat to guarantee self preservation and subsistence in the long term, with generalized health damage.

4.4 BROWN FAT TISSUE

*T*he basic rate of body fat burning depends on genetic factors, physical exercise levels, and body hormonal relations. However, some people expends calories in a much easier way than others. The body possesses an extra mechanism for expending calories, which helps determine our tendency to be lean or fat. Our body possesses a special kind of tissue called *brown fat tissue*, or *brown fat*, localized mainly behind the neck and along our dorsal spine, that helps in the release of extra calories. The brownish color is due to the high concentration of *mitochondria*, small units of energy production inside the cells. The brown fat tissue burns caloric nutrients only for heat production (thermogenesis) and not to produce energy for body movements (work). One of the functions of brown fat is weight stabilization and another is adaptation to cold climates.

Our appetite control is centered in a region of the brain called *hypothalamus* (our primitive brain, that also controls body temperature and other autonomic functions). The regulation of appetite uses a feedback mechanism that samples the amounts of insulin and amino acids (proteins) present in the bloodstream. Evidences indicate that the hypothalamus can activate brown fat to release extra calories every time excessive food intake occurs. Obese people that have difficulty losing weight probably have insufficient amounts of brown fat or a defective mechanism for activation of this tissue (and possibly a hormonal unbalance). The *gamma-linolenic* fatty acid (GLA) plays an important

> The brown fat tissue has a high concentration of mitochondria for extra release of calories, or thermogenesis.

role in the stimulation of the brown fat tissue, producing some prostaglandins that accelerate the mitochondria activity in this tissue, helping to lose weight. Prostaglandins are substances similar to hormones (chemical messengers), but of short reach and duration, that control a series of important functions in the body cells and tissues (these substances are described in the chapter on fatty acids and health).

4.5 EXCESS INSULIN AND AGING

Insulin is a hormone essential to life when present in normal levels, but when in excess it is extremely harmful. Excess insulin is a potential enemy that can cause high blood levels of glucose, triglycerides, and cholesterol, low levels of the high-density lipoprotein (HDL, popularly known as good cholesterol), hypertension, and may lead to the development of atherosclerosis, cellular damage, diabetes, precocious aging, and premature death. It is essential to normalize the blood levels of insulin in order to avoid all those problems.

Excess insulin accelerates glycation and free-radical activity, and stimulates the growth of smooth muscle cells on the artery walls, in which fatty plaques tend to accumulate, hardening and narrowing the arteries, which reduces blood flow (atherosclerosis). It also interferes with the system of blood clot formation and dissolution, which may result in arterial obstruction. Atherosclerosis shortens the lifespan, and it develops among people whose eating consists, largely, of refined carbohydrates, such as products that contain sugars and white flour (and sometimes with addition of hydrogenated vegetable oils, or vegetable fats, that contain trans-fat antinutrients).

High triglyceride blood levels are also associated with low blood levels of the high-density lipoprotein (HDL, good cholesterol). This lipoprotein helps in the removal of excess cholesterol eventually left in the tissues by the low-density lipoprotein (LDL, popularly known as bad cholesterol), transporting the excess to other tissues that may need cholesterol, or to the liver for remodeling. Insulin excess increases the liver production of LDL and stimulates the production of smaller and denser LDL particles, considered potentially harmful to the cardiovascular system. The blood lipoproteins and cholesterol are analyzed in detail in the chapters on cholesterol.

Hyperinsulinism is normally associated with insulin resistance and excess blood glucose. Glucose intolerance may lead to type 2 diabetes mellitus. It is also one of the causes of hypertension, causing the blood vessels to contract, increasing the blood pressure. Excess glucose leads also to the production of AGEs (Advanced Glycosylation End Products) that occur when the additional glucose in the system combines with the proteins in the body, damaging the tissue cells and causing premature aging. Excess insulin also promotes the growing of cancer cells.

> Cell resistance to insulin and hyperinsulinism cause excess blood levels of glucose and lead to premature aging.

4.6 NORMALIZING YOUR INSULIN LEVELS

*T*o maintain healthy insulin levels in the blood, it is essential to avoid sugar (in all its forms), refined carbohydrates, and high-GI carbohydrates, as well as to restrict the ingestion of sweet fruits and fruit juices rich in fructose. It is advisable not to ingest carbohydrates in excess, even whole unprocessed grains, as the need for insulin will still be high. Experts also recommend avoiding ingestion of refined vegetable oils that are highly susceptible to oxidation (such as industrially refined soy, corn, and sunflower oils), hydrogenated vegetable oils (such as margarine and vegetable fats that contain trans fats), and deep fried foods, which fills the bloodstream with free radicals potentially harmful to the cells. In the absence of sufficient amounts of antioxidant vitanutrients to neutralize the free radicals, these may exhaust some enzymes that help in glucose metabolism, resulting in the accumulation of glucose in the blood and extra insulin production in an attempt to metabolize the excess glucose. A more stable and safer type of fat is monounsaturated, present in olive oil, canola oil, avocados, nuts (e.g. macadamias), seeds, and peanuts.

Some researchers recommend the ingestion of chromium supplements (such as chromium picolinate), since the mineral increases insulin efficiency, so that the body will need less of this hormone to process glucose. Recommended daily dosages are of 200 micrograms. Vitamin E can also increase insulin efficiency, protecting the integrity of cell membranes against oxidative damage promoted by free radicals and reverting insulin resistance. The recommended daily dosage is at least 100UI and, preferably, 400UI. Losing weight also stimulates the normal insulin activity. The more body fat you have, the greater the insulin resistance.

To maintain healthy insulin blood levels we must avoid sugar, in all its forms, as well as refined and high-GI carbohydrates.

Large meals make your blood levels of glucose and insulin to increase drastically. It is much healthier to have several small meals distributed along the day. In other words, to nibble at healthy foods all day long is better than having three large meals per day. Keep in mind that proteins and good fats do not affect blood glucose levels directly, and, when consumed with some carbohydrates, they may actually decrease the carbohydrate glycemic index. There is evidence also that some herbs and spices (e.g. cinnamon) stimulate insulin efficiency, as well as the moderate consumption of alcoholic beverages, especially red wine (one to two drinks per day, maximum).

Also, it may be wise to avoid wheat and similar grains (seeds of grasses). Man evolved on a grain-free diet and wheat was only recently (during the last ten thousand years) introduced in the human diet. There are many adverse components in wheat and other similar cereal grains (like barley, rye, corn, oat, and rice) that have a negative effect on health. Consumption of wheat, while a global food staple usually believed to be healthy, is probably one of the worst mistakes in the history of the human race, due to some proteins (like gluten) and anti-nutrients that are allergenic, promote inflammation, compromise the immune system and digestive function, and promote systemic inflation. Wheat might be one of the most offensive foods in our diet that cause many health problems beyond just gaining weight or diabetes. Some researchers advocate that a wheat-free diet may greatly improve health (e.g. William Davis; Mark Sisson; see bibliography). Plants and animals (like meat, fish, fowl, eggs, cheese, vegetables, fruits, nuts and seeds) should be preferred in our diet.

4.7 IN SUMMARY

*F*oods that contain carbohydrates are normally classified by their glycemic index (GI), which measures the rate (or speed) at which their glucose enters the bloodstream after ingestion, and by their glycemic load (GL); see Tables 4.1 and 4.2. The best carbohydrate foods are those that have a low GI and a low GL, as for example yogurts (without sugar), soybeans, peanuts, beans, peas, nuts, and seeds.

Spaced and glycemic large meals make your glucose blood levels fluctuate drastically, stressing the pancreas and the adrenal glands. Try eating several small meals distributed along the day and avoid the ingestion of glycemic carbohydrates, especially at night.

To burn the fat stored in the body and to lose weight, experts recommend the following:

➢ Adequately limit the total of ingested calories, that is, your total daily calorie intake must be less, but not too much, than your total daily expended calories.
➢ Restrict the ingestion of carbohydrates, avoiding all the high-GI carbohydrates and limit yourself only to the consumption of low-GI whole carbohydrates, in controlled amounts.
➢ Choose a balanced diet that contains complete proteins and healthy fats, together with good sources of vitamins, minerals, and antioxidants.
➢ Practice physical exercise (without exaggeration), but respect your physical limitations.

The restriction of calories from carbohydrates allows for the burning of stored body fat, using it as an energy source. Supplements of L-carnitine and chromium help in this process. Also, it may be wise to avoid wheat and similar cereal grains.

> **TABLE 4.3 –** Calorie content and relative composition of macronutrients (in grams) in 100g of some foods that contain carbohydrates.

Note: **Cal** = Calories; **Carb** = Carbohydrate; **Prot** = Protein; **Fat** = Total fat;
    Sat = Saturated fat; **Unsat** = Unsaturated fat.

FRUITS	Cal	Carb	Prot	Fat	Sat	Unsat
Apple	55	14	0.2	0.3	0.1	0.2
Apricot	50	11.5	1.4	0.3	0	0.3
Avocado	160	7.5	2.0	15	2.5	12.5
Banana	95	24	1.1	0.5	0.2	0.3
Fig	70	18	0.8	0.3	0	0.3
Grape (green)	50	13	0.5	0.1	0	0.1
Grape (red)	70	14	1.3	1	0	1
Guava	50	12	0.8	0.5	0.2	0.3
Kiwi	60	15	1.0	0.4	0.1	0.3
Lemmon	30	9	1.0	0.3	0	0.3
Mango	65	17	0.5	0.3	0	0.3
Nectarine	45	11	0.9	0.4	0.1	0.3
Orange	45	12	0.9	0.2	0	0.2
Papaya	40	10	0.6	0.1	0	0.1
Peach	45	12	0.7	0.1	0	0.1
Pear	60	15	0.4	0.4	0.1	0.3
Pinapple	50	12	0.4	0.4	0.1	0.3
Plum	55	14	0.8	0.6	0.1	0.5
Strawberry	30	7	0.6	0.4	0	0.4
Tangerine	45	11	0.6	0.2	0	0.2
Tomato	20	4	0.9	0.2	0	0.2
Watermelon	35	8	0.6	0.4	0.1	0.3

(Cont.)

(Cont.)

CEREALS AND VEGETABLES	Cal	Carb	Prot	Fat	Sat	Unsat
Beans	130	23	9	0.5	0.1	0.4
Beet	31	7	1.1	0	0	0
Broccoli	30	5	3	0.2	0	0.2
Carrot	45	10	1	0.1	0	0.1
Corn	110	26	3.3	1.3	0.3	1.0
Egg-plant	30	7	0.8	0.2	0	0.2
Manioc	350	86	0.2	0	0	0
Onion	30	7	1	0.2	0	0.2
Pea	85	16	5.5	0.3	0	0.3
Potato	110	25	2.3	0.1	0	0.1
Soy	340	9	16	6.5	1	5.5
Spinach	25	3.3	3	0.2	0	0.2
Sweet potato	105	25	1.8	0.1	0	0.1
White rice	140	30	2.5	0.2	0.1	0.1
Whole rice	110	23	2.3	0.8	0.2	0.6

VARIOUS FOODS	Cal	Carb	Prot	Fat	Sat	Unsat
Beer (350ml/350g)	155	14	1	0	0	0
Bread (hamburger)	285	50	8.5	5	0	5
Bread (white)	280	50	8.3	3.8	0	3.8
Bread (whole)	245	44	9.5	4.4	0	4.4
Brewer´s yeast	290	40	40	1	0	1
Cacau powder (no sugar)	390	50	22	11	7	4
Chocolate bar	535	57	7	30	16	14
Chocolate bar (white)	535	53	10	33	20	13
Chocolate bar (with nuts)	560	50	10	36	20	16
Chocolate cookiet	535	67	0	27	14	13
Condensed milk	335	57	7	8	5	3
Condensed milk (without fat)	265	60	10	0	0	0
Corn biscuit	490	57	7	26	0	26
Corn flakes	395	86	8.2	0.4	0	0.4
Corn starch	365	88	0	0	0	0

(Cont.)

(Cont.)

VARIOUS FOODS	Cal	Carb	Prot	Fat	Sat	Unsat
Cracker (cream)	425	65	10	15	12	3
Cracker (water and salt)	480	76	10	15	6	9
Cracker (whole)	435	63	10	16	6	10
Cracker (with sesame)	435	60	8	17	4	13
Macaroni	140	29	4.8	0.7	0.1	0.6
Milk powder (whole)	500	39	26	27	15	12
Milk powder (without fat)	350	55	35	0	0	0
Oat flakes	370	73	19	1.5	0.3	1.2
Oat bran	270	71	20	7.9	1.8	6.1
Popcorn	385	79	12.8	5	0.7	4.3
Pretzels	370	77	8.8	3.4	0.8	2.6
Rice flakes	400	89	6.8	0.7	0	0.7
Spaghetti	140	29	4.8	0.6	0.1	0.5
Wheat flour (white)	365	80	8	0.8	0	0.8
Wheat flour (whole)	340	72	14	1	0	1
Wheat germ	385	54	29	11	1.8	9.2
Yogurt with fruits	115	21	3.3	2.5	1.7	0.8
Yogurt with fruits (no fat)	60	10	3.3	0	0	0

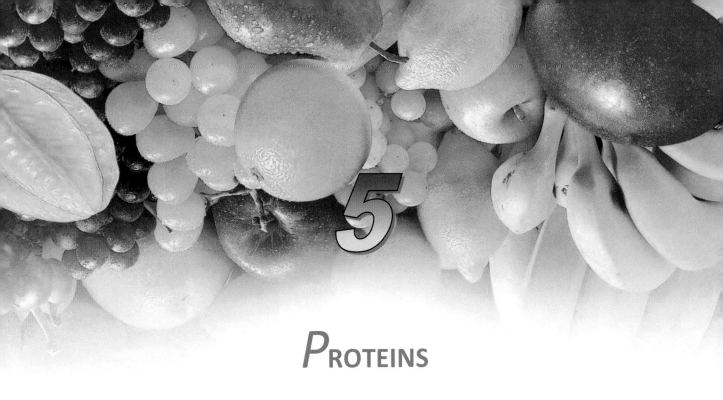

PROTEINS

AND AMINO ACIDS

5.1 MACROMOLECULES FOR BODY CONSTRUCTION

Proteins are the most abundant substances in our body, after water, being fundamental for health maintenance and for the development of all body components. They are, functionally, versatile biological macromolecules that constitute the main raw material for the construction of practically all body tissues, including bones, nerves, muscles, blood, skin, hair, nails, connective tissues, and internal organs, including the heart and the brain, and they perform myriads of other tasks. Many substances necessary for vital functions are also proteins, such as blood hemoglobin, elastin and collagen (formed of fibrous structures of proteins), some hormones (as insulin and glucagon, secreted by the pancreas), antibodies (imunoglobins for body defense), and enzymes (substances that act as catalysts, or reaction-promoting substances, in all biochemical reactions involved in body metabolism).

Besides being the main source of matter for body construction, proteins can also be used as an energy source (supplying about 4.3 calories per gram), when enough amounts of carbohydrates or fats are not present. Excess protein that is not used for tissue build up, or as energy, may also be converted by the liver and stored as body fat, for subsequent use as energy. As the body cannot store proteins in their original form, they need to be ingested daily.

> Proteins are versatile biological macromolecules that constitute the main raw material for the construction of all body tissues.

During digestion, the food protein macromolecules are broken into smaller molecules, called *amino acids*, which constitute the building blocks of all proteins. These amino acids are necessary, in certain relative proportions, for the synthesis of all body proteins. They are the basic units from which all the various proteins in the body are synthesized, and they are the final products of food protein digestion. Most protein chains contain some hundreds of amino acids in their molecule.

For each protein molecule in our body there exists a cellular *DNA segment* (a *gene*) that codifies the sequence of amino acids of this protein. In a typical cell, there are thousands of different proteins, where each one performs a specific function and each one is codified by a certain gene. Therefore, the genetic information is ultimately expressed as molecular structure of body proteins.

5.2 ESSENTIAL AMINO ACIDS

*O*ur body requires twenty basic amino acids, chemically combined in specific patterns, to produce the protein molecules that influence and define each cell of the body. Of these amino acids, nine are *essential*, in the sense that they cannot be synthesized by the body, even though they are fundamental for good health, so that they must be obtained from food

> The body cannot store proteins in their original form and they need to be ingested daily.

sources. The other amino acids, denominated *nonessential* (but as important as the essential ones), can be synthesized by the body, starting from other biochemical components, if the necessary raw material is available.

The nine essential amino acids are:

Methionine (Met), Threonine (Thr), Tryptophan (Trp), Leucine (Leu), Isoleucine (Ile), Lysine (Lys), Valine (Val), Phenylalanine (Phe), and Histidine (His).

> Amino acids are the basic building blocks of all proteins, in a sequence codified by a cellular DNA segment (a gene).

The other eleven natural amino acids are:

Glycine (Gly), Alanine (Ala), Proline (Pro), Tyrosine (Tyr), Serine (Ser), Cysteine (Cys), Asparagine (Asn), Glutamine (Gln), Aspartic acid (Asp), Glutamic acid (Glu), and Arginine (Arg).

Histidine may be considered essential only in childhood. Sometimes a nonessential amino acid may become essential (and must be obtained from food) when biosynthesis is limited, due to special physiological conditions. Arginine is, in some cases, considered essential, also during childhood, when the body needs overwhelms the metabolic synthesis. In spite of the fact that the body metabolism synthesizes arginine, most of it is decomposed, forming urea and other metabolic products. These twenty

> Essential amino acids cannot be synthesized by the body. They are essential for good health and must be obtained from food.

amino acids constitute the building blocks of all proteins in the body, assembled in certain sequences or patterns, codified by the cellular DNA segments.

5.3 BIOCHEMICAL CHARACTERISTICS OF PROTEINS

*P*roteins, in their basic chemical element composition, differ from carbohydrates and lipids. Besides carbon (C), hydrogen (H), and oxygen (O), their molecules invariably contain nitrogen (N) and, sometimes, the mineral sulfur (S). The simplest amino acid is *glycine*, whose chemical formula is shown in Figure 5.1, for illustrative purposes. In the representation shown, the lines indicate chemical bonds, where carbon is tetravalent, nitrogen is trivalent, oxygen is bivalent, and hydrogen is monovalent. This formula can be written in a compact form as $H_2C(NH_2)COOH$.

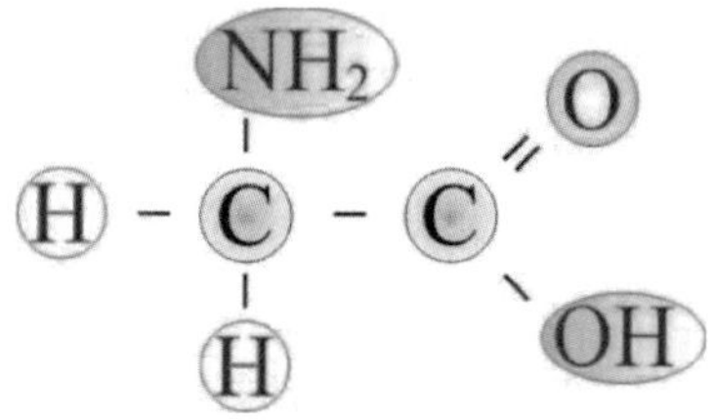

FIGURE 5.1 - Chemical formula of glycine, the simplest amino acid.

Other amino acids possess a larger number of carbon atoms in their carbon chain. *Alanine*, for instance, possesses the chemical formula $(CH_3)CH(NH_2)COOH$, the formula of *valine* is $(CH_3)_2CHCH(NH_2)COOH$ and the formula of *lysine* is $(NH_2)(CH_2)_4CH(NH_2)COOH$. In general (with the exception of *proline*), amino acids consist of a central carbon atom chemically bonded to one hydrogen atom, one *amino group* or radical $(-NH_2)$, one *carboxylic acid group* $(-COOH)$, and one side group that gives each amino acid its chemical identity.

The acidity characteristic of amino acids is conferred by the carboxylic acid group or radical $(-COOH)$. This group, together with the amino group or radical $(-NH_2)$, present in all amino acids, are fundamental in the formation of protein molecules. In aqueous solutions, the amino acids become ionized, in other words, they form *bipolar structures*, where the amino radical becomes a positive pole (NH_3^+) and the carboxylic acid radical becomes a negative pole (COO^-). This characteristic *acid-base* behavior is important to understand the biochemical properties of proteins. Amino acids can combine among themselves, forming larger chains, where the amino group of an amino acid bonds to the carboxylic group of another, forming connections that repeat themselves (called *peptide bonds*). In these reactions a water molecule (H_2O) is released, where the carboxylic acid group loses an oxygen atom and a

> In aqueous solutions the amino acids become ionized, presenting bipolar structures.

hydrogen atom, and the amino group loses a hydrogen atom. The resulting compounds of joined amino acids are denominated *peptides* and the polymeric molecular chains of peptides are called *polypeptides*. These amino acid polymeric chains occur biologically in many sizes, from small molecules, with only two (*dipeptides*) or three amino acids (*tripeptides*), up to large macromolecules with thousands of amino acids. Proteins in the body and in the diet are long polypeptides, most with hundreds of bonded amino acids.

A remarkable characteristic of the amino acids that form the protein molecules used in the body is that they are always of the *stereoisomeric* L form. The *spatial isomers* L (of *levo-rotation*, where *levo* means "left") and D (of *dextro-rotation*, where *dextro* means "right") constitute chemical compounds that

> Amino acids can bond chemically to each other in long polymeric molecular chains called polypeptides.

possess the same chemical formula, but differ in their spatial structure. They also possess different chemical properties. For illustrative purposes, it is shown in Figure 5.2 the chemical formula of the L and D stereoisomers of alanine, whose molecule structures present a spatial asymmetry in relation to the middle carbon atom (*chiral center*). The disposition of the atoms in the molecules of these two isomers presents spatial structures that are not superposable, similar to the right and left hands.

5.4 COMPLETE AND INCOMPLETE FOOD PROTEINS

*I*n order to synthesize the proteins that the body needs, the necessary amino acids, for each kind of protein, must be present, at the same time, in a proper relative proportion. In the case of a wrong, or incomplete, proportion, an insufficient amount of an amino acid will limit the protein biosynthesis by our metabolism, and the body will not be able to synthesize, in proper amounts, the proteins necessary for the muscles, skin, organs, and other tissues. When a food contains all the essential amino acids, in appropriate amounts, it is denominated a *complete protein*. A protein food in which one of the essential amino acids is absent, or present in minimum amounts, is called an *incomplete protein*.

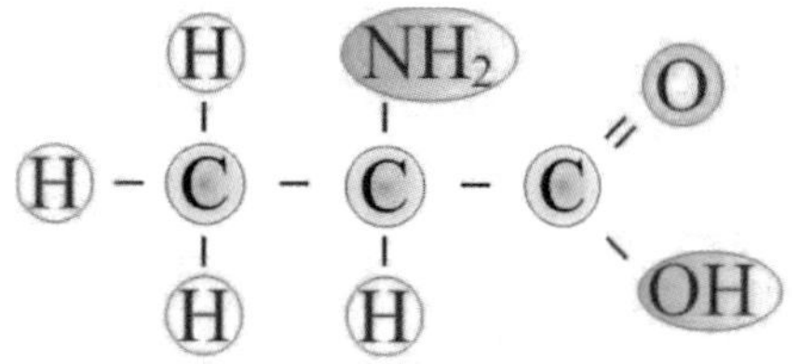

L-alanine 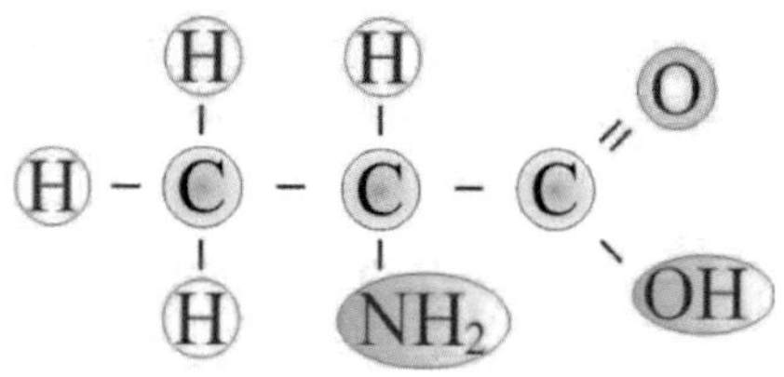   **D-alanine**

FIGURE 5.2 - The stereoisomers L and D of the amino acid alanine. Their spatial structures are non-superimposable images, similar to the right and left hands.

The proteins of *animal* origin, as the ones found in meats, poultry, fish, cheese, and eggs, normally contain all the essential amino acids necessary to the human body and, for this reason, they are considered *complete*. A given portion supplies all nine essential amino acids.

A complete food protein is one that contains all the essential amino acids in appropriate amounts.

Proteins of *vegetable* origin are denominated *incomplete*, because no vegetable or grain contains, in appropriate amounts, all nine essential amino acids simultaneously. Nevertheless, as the relative proportions of essential amino acids vary from one vegetable to another, there is the possibility to combine different vegetables, in a given meal, in order to produce a vegetarian diet that contains all nine essential amino acids simultaneously, in a reasonable relative proportion.

When a certain amount of a *nonessential* amino acid is lacking, the body is able to produce more, as long as the needed biochemical compounds are available. However, when deficiency of an *essential* amino acid occurs, the body metabolism cannot function properly, and, in cases of necessity, the body will begin to cannibalize its own muscular tissue, in order to extract the necessary essential amino acids. The body is continually being renewed, so that it needs complete proteins daily.

Animal proteins, as the ones contained in meats, poultry, fish, cheese, and eggs, are considered of *high quality* or *high biological value*, because they can provide all the essential amino acids in an appropriate relative proportion, and they are easily digested. Vegetables always lack one or more of the essential amino acids, or they don't have them in the necessary amounts, and are usually labeled as having a low index of protein efficiency. Many vegetarians that do not consume cheese and eggs are frequently in need of amino acid supplements. Soy protein, for instance, is deficient in the essential amino acids methionine and tryptophan.

A reasonably balanced amino acid combination in a high quality protein, for instance, is approximately the following (in 100g): valine, 11g; phenylalanine and tyrosine, 17g; leucine, 10g; amino acids that contain sulfur, 6g; lysine, 12g; threonine, 20g; tryptophan, 3g; isoleucine, 10g; and histidine, 4g. Table 5.1 shows the average values of the normal amino acid concentrations that are usually found in the blood serum as a function of age.

> The body is continually being renewed and it needs high-quality protein foods daily.

One of the most efficient sources of high quality food protein is the egg, which contains all the essential amino acids in an adequately balanced way. In fact, its relative amino acid proportion is the pattern usually used as base for the judgment of other protein sources. Eggs have been avoided, erroneously, in the last decades, because the yolk is rich in cholesterol. However, it is currently known that about 20% to 30% of the cholesterol present in the bloodstream comes from the diet and that the remaining part is produced by the liver, mainly from carbohydrates and fats (see the chapters on cholesterol). The liver produces, daily, about 2.5g to 3.5g of cholesterol. However, each person processes cholesterol according to his own biotype or genetic and biochemical individuality.

> Eggs are high-quality food proteins, rich in nutrients like lecithin, zinc, sulfur, choline, and important antioxidants.

TABLE 5.1 – Average values of normal amino acid concentrations (in μmol/liter) usually found in the bloodstream, as a function of age.

AMINO ACID	Newly-born	Toddlers	Children	Adults
Alanine (Ala)	329	292	234	360
β-alanine (Ala)	15	-	-	-
Arginine (Arg)	54	63	53	82
Asparagine (Asn)	8	19	10	-
Cysteine (Cys)	62	42	60	49
Glutamic Acid (Glu)	52	-	110	24
Glutamine (Gln)	-	-	-	640
Glycine Gly)	343	213	166	284
Histidine (His)	77	78	55	88
Hydroxyproline (Hyp)	32	-	25	-
Isoleucine (Ile)	39	39	43	60
Leucine (Leu)	72	77	85	115
Lysine (Lys)	200	135	111	186
Methionine (Met)	29	18	14	21
Ornitine (Orn)	91	50	33	58
Phenylalanine (Phe)	78	55	42	48
Proline (Pro)	183	193	106	185
Serine (Ser)	163	131	94	99
Taurine (Tau)	141	-	80	59
Threonine (Thr)	217	177	76	138
Tryptophan (Trp)	32	-	-	31
Tyrosine (Tyr)	69	54	43	54
Valine (Val)	136	161	162	225

Current research indicates that, for most people, a reduction in the ingestion of food cholesterol does not have a significant effect in their blood cholesterol concentration, because the body metabolism has a regenerative mechanism that reduces the rate of cholesterol synthesis when the ingestion is increased, and vice versa. Furthermore, eggs also contain lecithin (besides countless of other important body nutrients), that helps in the reduction of excessive cholesterol levels in many individuals (see the chapter on good fats and oils). Lecithin also acts as a fat emulsifier in the blood, preventing the formation of deposits or plaques on the artery walls. Eggs are also rich in nutrients like zinc, sulfur, choline, and important antioxidants (such as lutein and zeaxanthin).

Although a vegetarian diet may be rich in certain vitamins, carotenoids, antioxidants, fibers, and other protecting nutrients, it is usually deficient in some important nutrients, as vitamin B_{12} (available mainly from animal food sources) and some essential amino acids. A more beneficial form of vegetarian diet is one that includes, at least, eggs and milk derivatives (as cheese and yogurt).

5.5 DIFFERENT PROTEINS FOR DIFFERENT FUNCTIONS

*P*roteins are fundamental for muscle development, tissue growth, damaged tissue repair, production of enzymes, hormones, antibodies, hemoglobin, and collagen, and they play an important role in the formation of brain neurotransmitters. They allow the body to generate new cells to substitute those that die every day. Without enough proteins, new healthy cells cannot be formed, the skin (the body largest organ) may become dry and thin, hair becomes fragile and starts to fall, nails become brittle, muscular tone declines, and there may be muscular mass loss.

The body contains thousands of different proteins that serve many different purposes, and they must be renewed continually. Nails, hair, and the outer layer of the skin consist of the protein *keratin*, while muscles are constituted of protein fibers called *myosin* and *actin*. *Collagen* is a fibrous protein that strengthens the veins, blood arteries, skin, bones, teeth, and the intercellular cement (which unites the cells of tissues and organs). The globular proteins dissolved in the blood act as enzymes to promote and accelerate many biochemical reactions essential to life. *Hemoglobin* (the blood red cells globular protein) transports oxygen molecules from the lungs to all parts of the body, being

> The body contains thousands of different proteins that serve many different purposes and they must be renewed continually.

essential for energy production through the burning of metabolic fuels.

Proteins are made of long chains of amino acids and their nature is determined by the sequence of those amino acids in the polypeptide chain. Hemoglobin, for instance, consists of four peptide chains, two of which have 140 amino acids each and the other two have 146 amino acids each. Besides the sequence of amino acids in the polymeric chains, proteins are also characterized by the spatial disposition (three-dimensional structure) of their amino acids. Every protein has a unique three-dimensional structure that reflects its function in the body. In hair, the keratin chains are spiraled in the form of a spring. In a globular protein (as the hemoglobin or the digestive enzyme trypsin) there are straight and spiral segments, but the chain bends in an almost spherical structure. In silk, the amino acid chains are linearly disposed. The sequence of amino acids for similar proteins (same biological function) in different animals is also different.

There are normally four levels of recognized protein structure or three-dimensional configurations. The *primary structure* refers to the sequence of amino acids and the location of the so-called disulfit bridges. The *secondary structure* refers to the spatial relationship of adjacent amino acids. The *tertiary structure* is a three-dimensional conformation of the whole polypeptide chain. The *quaternary structure* refers to the spatial relationship of multiple polypeptide chains. Collagen, for instance, possesses a structure in the form of a repetitive triple helix (a secondary structure).

> Proteins are made of long chains of amino acids and their nature is determined by the sequence of amino acids in the polypeptide chain.

5.6 PROTEINS AND BODY METABOLISM

The rate at which the body burns stored fat is closely related to the amount of body lean muscular mass. The greater the body lean muscular mass, the greater the metabolic rate, and more calories will be burned daily. Protein is fundamental for the formation of muscles and, consequently, to increase the rate at which the body burns stored fat. Therefore, to produce lean muscular mass and to accelerate the metabolic rate to burn stored fat it is necessary to ingest enough amounts of complete proteins. On the other hand, insufficient ingestion of protein leads to muscular mass loss, reduction in the metabolic rate, and increase in the rate of fat accumulation.

An important function of proteins is to stimulate the pancreas to produce the hormone *glucagon.* Glucagon responds to low blood sugar content and increases the rate at which glycogen in the liver is broken down to glucose. One of its primary functions is to liberate the fat stored in the cells to be used as energy. Excess of the *insulin* hormone in the blood (usually caused by an excessive ingestion of simple carbohydrates of high glycemic index) inhibits the production of glucagon, impeding the liberation of stored fat. Consequently, the body is not able to burn its own fat. The ingestion of appropriate amounts of protein (in combination

> Proteins stimulate the pancreas to produce the hormone glucagon, which helps body metabolism to burn stored fat.

with healthy lipids and restriction of glycemic carbohydrates), stimulates the pancreas to produce enough glucagon to liberate the fat stored in the cells, allowing the body to burn excess fat for energy production. Thus, proteins act in the opposite sense of insulin, stabilizing blood glucose levels and supplying the body with a more steady energy flow.

Proteins also strengthen the immune system, contributing to antibody production, the corporal agents that fight diseases and infections caused by virus and/or bacteria. It is essential for the healthy operation of *leucocytes* and *lymphocytes* (white cells present in blood and lymphatic vessels), helping to maintain a healthy cellular metabolism and an efficient resistance to bacteria and other invaders.

Another function of proteins is the maintenance of proper body fluid balance, with the help of some minerals. Proteins in the blood control

> Insufficient protein intake leads to muscular mass loss, reduction in metabolic rate, and increase in body fat accumulation.

the aqueous levels between cells, inside cells, and inside arteries and veins. A low-protein diet affects this fluid balance and, consequently, the efficient elimination of fluids by the kidneys, which could result in retention of water in the body.

5.7 HISTORICAL RELEVANCE OF PROTEINS

Through time, human beings have obtained their food from sources of both animal origin (such as meats, poultry, fish, eggs, milk, and milk derivatives) and vegetable origin (such as nuts, seeds, fruits, legumes, cereals, leaves, and other vegetables). Food protein from animal sources has been a fundamental component of human nutrition for many thousands of years. Although, for us, this may seem like a long time, for human genetics it is actually little in the historical evolution process. Any difference that may exist between our present genetic structure and that of the human beings that lived in the Paleolithic era, about 40,000 years ago, should be small. From a point of view of the human biology, the present processed foods (deprived of important nutrients, and rich in simple glycemic carbohydrates and artificially hydrogenated vegetable fats), are novelties to our body, and have been introduced only recently along the last century.

> Food protein from animal sources has been a fundamental component of human nutrition for many thousands of years.

In the last few decades, two of the best alimentary sources of complete proteins, namely meats and eggs, have been avoided and blamed for the occurrence of health problems such as high blood cholesterol levels, cardiovascular diseases, and obesity. Many people, in their phobia for foods that contain animal fat, eliminated from their diet good sources of complete proteins. It is known today that this is a serious mistake. The trans fats (present in partially hydrogenated vegetable oils or vegetable fats) incorporated in many industrialized and processed foods, play a much more significant role to increase the risk of heart disease than any other type of fat.

The evidence accumulated along the last decades indicates that the decrease in the consumption of natural foods rich in complete proteins and nutrients, and the increase in the consumption of sugars, refined carbohydrates, margarine, and processed foods caused a notable increase in the occurrence of cardiovascular diseases, obesity, and diabetes. It is now believed that the risks related to animal fat (mostly saturated) consumption were overestimated. Animal or saturated fat becomes harmful only when consumed excessively, together with unbalanced diets rich in simple (or refined) glycemic carbohydrates and processed foods containing vegetable fats, but not when consumed in moderation from foods rich in complete proteins and nutrients, and as part of a balanced diet.

Table 5.2 shows the relative composition of macronutrients in some protein-rich foods. Tables that contain the nutritional composition of thousands of foods can be found at the web site of the US Department of Agriculture (*http://www.ars.usda.gov/ba/bhnrc/ndl*).

TABLE 5.2 – Relative average composition of macronutrients (in grams) and calories of some protein-rich foods (per 100g).

Note: **Cal** = Calories; **Carb** = Carbohydrates; **Prot** = Proteins; **Fat** = Total fat; **Sat** = Saturated fat; **Unsat** = Unsaturated fat.

POULTRY	Cal	Carb	Prot	Fat	Sat	Unsat
Chicken: Dark meat	210	0	28	10	3	3
White meat	175	0	31	5	1.5	1
Heart	190	0	27	8	2.5	2.5
Liver	160	1	25	6	2	1
Turkey: Dark meat	190	0	29	7	3	2
White meat	160	0	30	3	1	1
Duck	200	0	24	11	4	1.5

FISH	Cal	Carb	Prot	Fat	Sat	Unsat
Anchovy, oil packed	210	0	29	10	2	7
Cod	100	0	23	1	0.2	0.5
Crab	120	0	19	1.5	0.2	0.7
Flounder	120	0	30	1	0.3	0.3
Grouper	120	0	25	1.3	0.4	0.4
Herring	200	0	23	9	2	6
Lobster	120	1	20	1	0.2	0.5
Salmon	200	0	24	7	1.5	5
Sardines, oil packed	200	0	25	11	1.5	9
Shark	130	0	21	4.5	1	3
Shrimp	110	0	21	1.5	0.2	1
Swordfish	150	0	25	2	0.5	1
Trout	150	0	26	4	1	2
Tuna, oil packed	200	0	25	10	2	7
Tuna, water packed	150	0	25	5	1.5	3

(cont.)

(cont.)

MEAT						
Beef: Ground beef, lean	270	0	24	18	7	9
Ground beef	300	0	25	22	9	10
Lean meat	270	0	22	19	8	9
Fat meat	320	0	28	24	10	11
Sirloin steak	300	0	26	21	8	9
Tenderloin	270	0	25	18	7	8
Pork: Bacon	540	0	29	48	17	28
Leg	300	0	25	22	9	8
Loin chop	230	0	23	19	7	10

CHEESE	Cal	Carb	Prot	Fat	Sat	Unsat
Blue	355	3	22	29	19	10
Camembert	305	0	20	25	16	9
Cheddar	405	0	25	34	22	12
Cottage	85	2	17	0.4	0.3	0.1
Cream	353	3	8	35	22	11
Edam	360	0	25	28	18	9
Gouda	360	3	25	28	18	10
Gruyere	420	0	30	33	20	13
Mozzarella	285	2	20	22	13	9
Parmesan	395	2	36	26	17	9
Parmesan, grated	460	0	40	30	20	10
Provolone	355	3	26	27	17	10
Ricotta	175	3	12	13	9	4
Roquefort	375	3	22	31	20	11
Swiss	380	3	29	28	18	10

(cont.)

(cont.)

EGG	Cal	Carb	Prot	Fat	Sat	Unsat
Chicken: Whole (100g)	160	2	12	11	3.5	6
White (100g)	51	1	11	0	0	0
Yolk (100g)	370	4	15	32	10	18
Chicken (one egg):						
Whole (50g)	80	1	6	5.5	1.7	3
White (33g)	17	0.3	3.5	0	0	0
Yolk (17g)	63	0.7	2.5	5.5	1.7	3
Duck: Whole (100g)	185	1.5	14	15	3.5	7.5

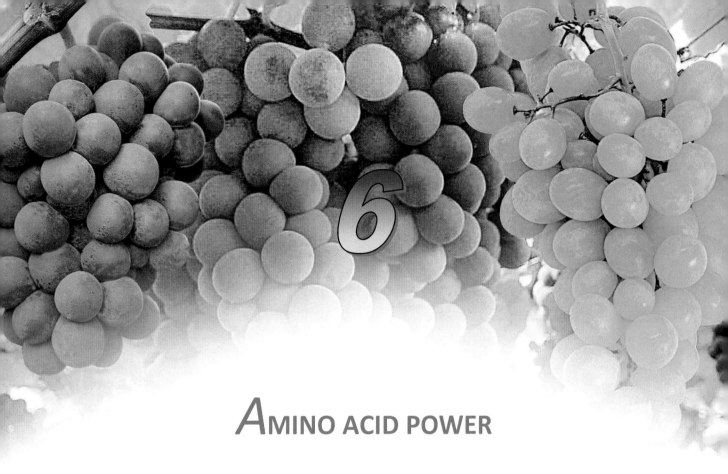

AMINO ACID POWER

6.1 FOOD PROTEIN DECOMPOSITION

*T*he food protein molecules that we ingest are too big and are unable to cross the intestinal walls in order to enter the bloodstream. During digestion in the stomach and in the small intestine, the digestive and pancreatic enzymes break the protein macromolecules into the component *amino acids*.

The *enzymes* (substances that catalyze the biochemical reactions) specialized in the decomposition of proteins are called *proteolytic enzymes* or *proteases*. The proteolytic enzymes are also known as peptidases, because they act on the polypeptidic chain that forms the skeleton or structure of proteins. More than twenty different peptidases are known to exist in the human body, and each one acts on a specific protein or on a certain class of proteins. Those enzymes disassemble the protein structure through a process called *hydrolysis* (where the suffix

During digestion, proteolytic enzymes decompose the protein macromolecules into amino acids, through a process called hydrolysis.

lysis means "to destroy"), in which water molecules are introduced in the polypeptidic chain, breaking it into amino acids. Pepsin, present in the stomach gastric juice, is a proteolytic enzyme that functions better in the stomach acidity created by the hydrochloric acid. In the small intestine, the enzymes in the pancreatic juice, as trypsin and quimotrypsin, complete the food protein decomposition into simpler polypeptide chains and, finally, into free amino acids that are absorbed in the blood through the intestinal walls.

In the cells, amino acids from food digestion are united again in long chains, obeying the characteristic sequences of human proteins dictated by the genetic code.

Those small amino acid molecules are transported through the blood to the various body tissues. After entering the cells, the amino acids are united again in long chains, obeying the characteristic sequences of human proteins. This process is performed according to the code contained in the *Deoxyribonucleic Acid* (or DNA), in the nuclei of the tissue cells, determining the nature of each protein. Some hormones interfere regularly in the reception of amino acids at the cells.

The proteins in the body, as well as other body molecules, are continually decomposed and rebuilt, in an endless process. The proteins introduced by food are decomposed and integrated with the ones in the body. At the same time, tissue proteins are also decomposed and rebuilt. Those transformations create a nitrogen reserve (or *metabolic nitrogen pool*) used in the reconstruction of proteins. Several experiments confirm the permanent exchange among the ingested proteins and those present in the body tissues. Our body is, therefore, continually rebuilding itself. The blood red cells, for instance, live for about just one month. When discarded, they are broken into the component amino acids.

For the reconstruction of body proteins it is important to maintain a positive metabolic nitrogen pool or reserve.

Some are used in the formation of new protein molecules, but some are oxidized (used as metabolic fuel), resulting in carbon dioxide, water, and urea (containing nitrogen). These last two are eliminated in the urine. For the formation of body proteins, it is important to maintain in the body a metabolic nitrogen pool (in other words, when the ingested nitrogen exceeds the excreted nitrogen), particularly during growth (children and adolescents), pregnancy, and recuperation.

6.2 PROPERTIES OF ESSENTIAL AMINO ACIDS

Phenylalanine. This amino acid plays an important role in healthy brain function and in the production of neurotransmitters, which are substances responsible for the alert state and for a positive mental disposition. Phenylalanine participates in the production of the chemical messengers (hormones) dopamine, epinephrine, and norepinephrine, involved in signal transmission through the nervous system. This amino acid helps in the relief of pain, including arthritis and menstrual colic. Some studies have shown that phenylalanine acts as an effective antidepressant and as an eliminator of pains in the brain. This amino acid is found mainly in meats, eggs, cheeses, wheat germ, almonds, peanuts, bananas, and avocados, for instance. People who have the genetic defect of severe mental retardation called PKU, or phenilketonuria (an inherited metabolic disease), should avoid foods that contain phenylalanine.

Histidine. Appropriate supplies of histidine regenerate and repair the body tissues. It is also a precursor of histamine, an active neurotransmitter in immunological response. Medicines for nasal allergies, or antihistamines, neutralize the histamines that this amino acid allows the organism to produce. It is necessary for the production of the red and white blood cells. The amino acid is necessary and essential for childhood growth, when the demand overwhelms the body's ability to produce it. Histidine is found mainly in meats, poultry, eggs, and cheeses.

Isoleucine. It is one of the three amino acids associated with tension or stress. Isoleucine is necessary for the production of hemoglobin and energy. Together with leucine and valine (the other two amino acids associated with stress), they are known as *branched-chain amino acids* (BCAAs). Good isoleucine sources are meats, poultry, eggs, cheeses, and some fish.

Leucine. Another amino acid associated with tension or stress. It is fundamental for growth, for bone and muscle construction, and for skin development. It is found in large concentrations mainly in lean muscle tissues. Meats, poultry, cheeses, and wheat germ are excellent leucine sources.

Lysine. This essential amino acid is particularly important for the health and development of skin, collagen, and bones, allowing the body to process calcium efficiently. Consequently, it is important in the control of osteoporosis. It also constitutes an effective form of treatment for herpes. Besides meats, poultry, eggs, cheeses, and fish, lysine is also abundant in some vegetables.

Methionine. This amino acid contains sulfur in its molecule. Methionine is critical for fat metabolism and acts as an antioxidant for the whole body. There is evidence that it aids in the relief of mental depression, inflammation, hepatic disease, and some muscular pains, and exerts a protection action to the liver. It is considered necessary for an effective use of the amino acids cysteine and taurine by the body. Good food sources are meats, eggs, cheeses, and, in smaller proportion, several nuts and seeds. Vegetarians need to provide an appropriate ingestion of methionine, because only minimum amounts of this amino acid exist in vegetables, including soybeans.

Threonine. It is fundamental for a healthy operation of the immune system. It also promotes the production of skin, bones, and teeth enamel, and supports a healthy functioning of the thymus gland (that controls the immune system). Food sources rich in threonine are meats, eggs, and vegetables (beans, soybeans, and peanuts).

Thryptophan. It is a precursor of serotonine, one of the chemical substances that regulate the transmission of nervous pulses to the brain. This neurotransmitter affects vitality, state of mind, behavior, and sleep functioning. Thryptophan relieves depression, calms anxiety, and helps allow a sound sleep. The well-known antidepressive drug Prozac, for instance, works by enhancing the serotonine levels in the brain. Thryptophan is found mainly in meats, poultry (especially turkey), cheeses, and nuts. Grains and vegetables are not important sources of thryptophan.

Valine. It is one of the three branched-chain amino acids associated with tension or stress, being fundamental for energy production. It contributes to the production of the growth hormones and is important for body metabolism.

6.3 PROPERTIES OF NONESSENTIAL AMINO ACIDS

Sometimes, for health maintenance, to cure a disease, or to improve athletic performance, the body may need amino acids in amounts and combinations that food cannot supply. Amino acids influence almost all body functions, preventing and curing several physical and mental diseases. Our body can manufacture nonessential amino acids starting from other biochemical compounds, but only in amounts limited to the availability of the necessary raw material, which may be insufficient or inexistent. Supplements of certain amino acids can naturally contribute to the maintenance of a good health.

> Amino acids can naturally influence body functions and help prevent or cure various physical and mental diseases.

The main functions of some important amino acids present in the body are described next. The letter L, preceding the name of the amino acid, refers to the levo-rotation stereoisomeric form, in opposition to the dextro-rotation stereoisomeric form, D. Only the L stereoisomeric form of amino acids is used by the body.

Glutamine. It is the most abundant amino acid in the body and, possibly, the most important. It is a derivative of glutamic acid. Glutamine possesses an extra nitrogen atom in its molecule, which can be used for the synthesis of other amino acids necessary for good recovery of several types of diseases. It helps the body to produce other important nutrients, such as glutathione, glucosamine, and vitamin B_3 (niacin). It maintains the structural integrity of the intestines, accelerates the healing of wounds and burns, and constitutes the main energy source for the immune system. It is, also, the largest energy source for the brain and an important piece for production of several neurotransmitters. This amino acid stimulates the pituitary gland to liberate the human growth hormone (HGH) that promotes muscular growth and delays, after middle age, the aging process. Supplements of L-glutamine constitute a simple and economical way to take this amino acid, being suggested about a teaspoon (5g) a day. To stimulate the secretion of HGH (human growth hormone) by the pituitary gland, it should be taken preferably at night.

Carnitine. This amino acid compound helps in the conversion of blood fat into fuel. It is not found in vegetable sources. Carnitine is necessary for the introduction of fat molecules (coming from triglycerides) into the cell mitochondria (small structures inside the cells, where elementary fuel oxidation occurs) for metabolic burning, supplying energy for muscular activity. The heart depends completely on carnitine, and two-thirds of its energy supply comes from the fats that carnitine allows the body to burn. This amino acid can protect the heart muscle from any possible damage, in case of infarct. It also elevates the levels of certain enzymes necessary for the metabolism of sugars, starches, and other carbohydrates. It is an important complement in any effort for body fat and weight loss, and to enhance physical resistance and muscular force. Carnitine can be synthesized by the body starting from the essential amino acids lysine and methionine, together with other nutrients as vitamin B_3, vitamin B_6, and iron. Appropriate ingestion of vitamin C helps to increase the amount of L-carnitine synthesized starting from lysine and methionine. Since it is one of the most necessary nutrients, to compensate possible deficiencies and for preventive purposes, specialists recommend supplements in quantities ranging from 500mg to 1g of L-carnitine per day. As most amino acids, L-carnitine is rarely toxic, even when ingested in large quantities.

Branched-Chain Amino Acids. L-leucine, L-isoleucine, and L-valine, also known as branched-chain amino acids (BCAAs), protect and preserve all muscles and tissues, except bones and fatty tissues. For this reason, athletes and those involved in heavy muscular activity and weight lifting have been using BCAA supplements. For good therapeutic effects, these three essential amino acids should be taken together with L-glutamine. According to research, everyone can benefit from BCAA supplements. The suggested therapeutic doses range from 3g to 4g of L-leucine, 2g to 3g grams of L-isoleucine, 4g to 5g of L-valine, and 4g to 6g of L-glutamine, per day.

Arginine. This amino acid stimulates the immunological system and is a precursor of nitric oxide (NO), considered a central piece for blood vessel relaxation and for the control of high blood pressure (not to be confused with nitrous oxide N_2O, known as laughing gas). This amino acid is considered of great value in cardiology. It can improve heart health, by inducing better coronary microcirculation in people with high blood cholesterol levels and preventing the formation of blood clots that can provoke infarcts and hemorrhages. Arginine also stimulates the body to produce the human growth hormone (HGH) and participates in the preservation of lean muscular tissues in the whole body. Supplements can reduce blood levels of the low-density lipoproteins (LDL, bad cholesterol) without reducing levels of the high-density ones (HDL, good cholesterol). Therapeutic doses can vary from 1.5g to 4g per day, as support to the immune system, and up to 15g per day, as part of cardiovascular therapy. Arginine supplements should be complemented with wide antioxidant protection (especially coenzyme Q_{10} and lipoic acid) to avoid the risk of arginine to stimulate oxidation by free radicals. People that suffer from arthritis, or from some active infection, should have caution with arginine supplements, because the excess nitric oxide may enhance the inflammation. Arginine is considered an essential amino acid during childhood, when its metabolic production is not sufficient to attend the body's needs.

Taurine. This amino acid compound contributes to the body antioxidant defenses. It reinforces the immune system, regulates the nervous system and the muscles, protects against diabetes, helps in digestion, strengthens the heart muscle, regulates heart contractions, and prevents the formation of clots. It also exerts diuretic function, through a control of the flow of some vitanutrients through the cellular membranes, maintaining potassium and magnesium inside the cells and sodium excess outside. Taurine helps to stabilize glucose levels in the blood, reinforcing cellular sensitivity to insulin. Our body can produce taurine starting from amino acids that contain sulfur, as cysteine and methionine, found in egg yolks and meats. However, in some conventional low-fat and low-protein diets (inadequate), these raw materials are usually scarce and supplements may be necessary.

Glutathione. This amino acid is the most abundant antioxidant enzyme in the body. Glutathione is also considered one of the most important body antioxidants and it is present inside and outside cells, protecting all cells, tissues, and organs. Its main function is to decompose and destroy toxins potentially noxious to the body, protecting it against lipid peroxidation. When not interrupted by antioxidant substances, lipid peroxidation damages the cells through a chain of oxidation reactions (also caused by all free radicals). Lack of glutathione in the cells is considered one of the causes of precocious aging. Glutathione disables countless carcinogenic substances, removes free radicals liberated by oxidized fat in the intestinal tract, and prevents blood cholesterol from becoming oxidized. Composed of three natural amino acids, it is found mainly in fresh fruits, vegetables, and meats, and it is also produced in the cells as part of their detoxication system. Our body manufactures glutathione starting from the amino acids cysteine, glycine, and glutamic acid, besides selenium and vitamins B_2 (riboflavin) and B_6 (pyridoxine). Supplements of L-glutamine stimulate the liver to synthesize glutathione, so that glutamine also constitutes a fantastic antioxidant and anti-aging agent.

Tyrosine. It is synthesized in the body starting from the essential amino acid phenylalanine, and it plays an important role in the production of three messengers (hormones) of the nervous system: dopamine, epinephrine, and norepinephrine. This amino acid acts as an excellent antidepressant. The neurotransmitters that help to deal with stress, as adrenalin and noradrenalin (which are produced by the adrenal gland), depend in great part on tyrosine. The larger the amount of tyrosine in the body, the better will be our condition to deal with stress and to avoid depression.

6.4 DIETARY PROTEIN SUPPLEMENTS

*T*here are high-quality protein supplements available commercially, obtained from natural sources, such as *milk whey, albumin* (egg white,) and soybeans, and also in the form of hydrolyzed peptides. Each protein type possesses a different amino acid profile. The proteins that are isolated and concentrated from milk whey are particularly rich in the three branched-chain amino acids L-leucine, L-isoleucine, and L-valine, known as BCAAs. Those obtained from albumin are rich in L-arginine and in amino acids that contain sulfur, such as L-cysteine and L-methionine. The hydrolyzed peptides are normally rich in L-glutamine, L-glutamic acid, and L-tryptophan. Supplements that combine multiple protein sources can provide excellent amino acid profiles.

> High-quality protein supplements can be used to complement a balanced diet.

6.5 MUSCLE ACTIVITY

*O*ur muscular tissues contain about 20% to 30% protein and their main function is to perform work (physical movements) using the energy liberated through the burning (oxidation) of elementary metabolic fuels. The muscles contract during performance and the contractile element is the protein *actomyosin* (composed of two fibrous proteins, *actin* and *myosin*). In the extended muscle, the tips of the actin molecule filaments just touch the tips of the myosin molecule filaments. During muscular contraction, the myosin filaments move through the channels between the actin filaments, attracted by specific intermolecular forces, accomplishing work.

The energy necessary for muscular contraction and movements comes from the burning or oxidation of some elementary nutrients (mainly glucose and lipids, and, sometimes, amino acids) inside the mitochondria, which are small structures inside the cells that act as small energy generation plants. After energy generation, the cells maintain a reserve in special energy-rich molecules called *adenosine triphosphate* (ATP), which liberates that energy when necessary. The burning of metabolic fuels in the mitochondria recharges the ATP molecules continually, using the phosphate contained in them for that purpose. The ATP molecules diffuse in the contracted muscle and liberate their energy, modifying the complementary structures of the actin and myosin filaments. That allows the muscle to relax and the protein filaments to return to their extended state, being ready to contract again when receiving a nervous impulse.

> Metabolic fuel burning in the interior of the cell mitochondria recharges the energy-rich molecules of adenosine triphosphate (ATP).

The amino acid *carnitine* is one of the orthomolecular substances involved in muscular activity, being necessary for the introduction of fatty acid molecules from the cytosol into the mitochondria, generating energy for the muscles. Only the stereoisomeric L form (levo-rotation) of carnitine, or L-carnitine, is effective in muscular activity. Supplements of L-carnitine may enhance muscular strength and athletic performance, and may help to decrease body fat.

6.6 DAILY PROTEIN INTAKE

People that suffer from protein deficiency can experience significant physical and emotional problems, such as muscular mass loss, body fat accumulation, deficient immune system, fatigue, mental confusion, depression, irritability, low libido, dry skin, brittle nails, weak hair, anemia, and liver diseases, among others. In the last few decades, many people eliminated from their diet some of the best protein sources, trying to reduce the ingestion of foods containing cholesterol, avoiding the consumption of fats in an indiscriminate way, and increasing the ingestion of foods rich in refined carbohydrates. Today, it is well known the inefficacy of this type of diet for the maintenance of a healthy body. Although it may be wise to avoid fatty meats and maturated meats, there seems to be no reasons to avoid lean meats, poultry, fish, eggs, and milk derivatives. They are excellent sources of protein and have many nutrients essential for healthy body functioning.

Recent research suggests that a diet with about 30% protein (relative to the total calories ingested) is ideal to promote a healthy organism and an efficient metabolism. Considering, for instance, a diet of 2,000 calories per day, this implies in about 150g of protein per day. This value is far superior to the minimum value recommended by American government organizations (about 1g of high quality protein per kilogram of body weight) for basic body maintenance. According to national survey data, the medium daily intake of protein for adult males range from 70g to 100g, which corresponds to about 1g to 1.5g of protein per kilogram weight, if we consider a reference body weight of 70kg. People with compromised renal function should limit their protein intake to the level of amino acids necessary for health maintenance.

It is important to point out that that an increase in protein consumption should be compensated by a corresponding decrease (in calories) in carbohydrate and fat consumption, in order to maintain a proper total calorie ingestion per day. Obviously, we should avoid sugar, refined carbohydrates, and foods with a high glycemic index, which affect blood glucose levels and insulin production. Also, we should avoid bad lipids, such as easily oxidized refined omega-6 vegetable oils, oils heated to high temperatures for long periods (as in fried foods), hydrogenated vegetable oils containing trans fats (as in margarine and some industrialized processed foods), and excess saturated fat consumption. Excess of amino acids, unnecessary to form new protein molecules, can be

> A diet with about 30% protein, relative to the total amount of calories ingested, is ideal to maintain a healthy body and an efficient metabolism.

eventually burned to generate energy, similar to carbohydrates and fats, or they may be reprocessed and converted into body fat in the case of an excessive ingestion of calories.

In general, large amounts of amino acids in the body are unlikely to cause any serious problems. However, the catabolism of amino acids yields some nitrogen compounds (due to the presence of nitrogen in the amino acid molecules), such as *urea*, that must be filtered from the blood by the kidneys and eliminated in the urine. Thus, large protein ingestion requires a higher renal activity in order for the kidneys to eliminate the extra amount of urea generated. Larger amounts of water should be consumed to stabilize this process. People with kidney deficiency or impaired renal function, for some reason, should avoid excessive intake of food protein and limit protein consumption to the necessary equilibrium level of amino acids in the body.

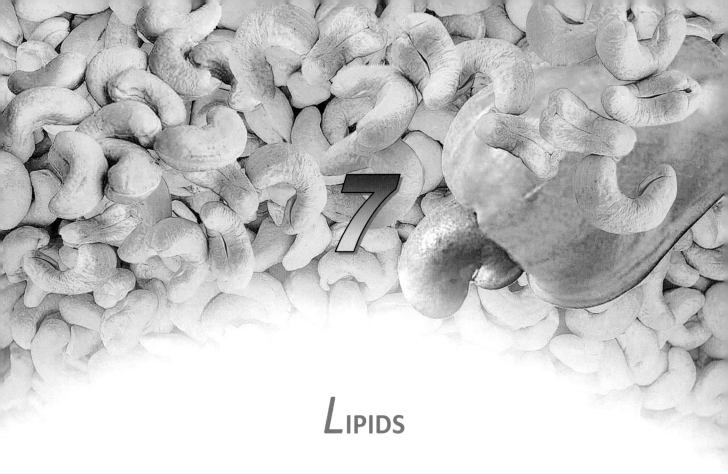

7

LIPIDS

7.1 CONCENTRATED ENERGY SOURCES

*T*he alimentary (nourishment) lipids, also known as *oils* or *fats*, are nutrients that supply energy for metabolic processes, maintain cell membranes and blood vessels, transmit nervous impulses, and produce essential hormones. They are necessary for the health of the brain and body. These substances are insoluble in water and slippery to the touch, and the many different types possess different biochemical properties. The lipids of interest in nutrition are generally classified in three types: *triglycerides*, *phospholipids*, and *sterols*. They represent the most concentrated energy source in foods (about 9kcal/g) when burned (oxidized) inside the cell mitochondria for energy production. The body can store fat provisions in the various tissues and under the skin layers for eventual use as energy sources.

The lipids are important functional and structural components of the body, and without them we would not survive. They supply energy for physical processes such as muscular functions, breathing, maintenance of tissues, and growth, and they also act in the conservation of body heat. They participate in body metabolism and in the transport of fat-soluble vitamins (A, D, E, and K) through the intestinal walls and into the bloodstream. Thus, they are essential for calcium absorption (which depends on vitamin D) by the tissues, bones, and teeth, and for the body antioxidant protection. They act in the conversion of cholesterol present in the skin into vitamin D (through the action of sunlight) and in the production of sexual hormones. Together with the mineral phosphorus (present in phospholipids), they participate in the formation of cellular membranes. They supply essential fatty acids (*linoleic, linolenic,* and *arachidonic acids*), which promote the growth of cells, tissues, and organs. The lipids are also fundamental ingredients for the production of *prostaglandins* (PGs), which are active substances similar to hormones but of short duration and reach, that control inflammatory processes, blood coagulation mechanisms, and blood arterial pressure, among others.

> The alimentary lipids are generally classified as triglycerides, phospholipids, and sterols. They are important functional and structural components of our body.

They act also as insulators to protect the nerves (such as the *myelin sheath*) and the muscles. They isolate and protect vital organs such as the heart, liver, kidneys, and glands, and they absorb impact during body movements. Foods become more palatable when mixed with oils and fats, which prolong the digestive process, diminish secretion of hydrochloric acid in the stomach, and give a feeling of satiety that lasts longer than with other foods such as carbohydrates. They also act as an intestinal lubricant.

7.2 FATTY ACIDS

The elementary substances that give lipids their different textures, flavors, melting temperatures, and biochemical properties are called *fatty acids*. The fatty acids are the chemical building blocks of lipids. The term *acid* refers to the chemical radical *carboxyl* (–COOH) of the lipid molecule (part soluble in water), and *fatty* refers to the chemical radical m*ethyl* (–CH₃) of the molecule (part not soluble in water). Essentially, the fatty acids are constituted of a carboxyl group bonded to a long hydrocarbon chain.

To understand the differences between the good lipids (that are fundamental for good health) and the bad lipids (that may be harmful) from a biochemical point of view, it is necessary to know some concepts used in the chemistry of lipids.

7.3 SATURATED AND UNSATURATED FATS

*F*atty acids differ in the length or size of their molecular carbon atom chain, which affects their absorption by the body, and in the type of *chemical bonds* (single or double) between the carbon atoms, that is, in the existence or not of double bonds between the carbon atoms in the hydrocarbon chain (*unsaturated* or *saturated*). The term *saturated* means that all carbon atoms in the hydrocarbon chain are bonded through single chemical bonds. Thus, all carbon atoms are saturated with hydrogen.

> Fatty acids are the chemical building blocks of lipids and are constituted of a carboxyl group bonded to a long hydrocarbon molecular chain.

For illustration purposes, a simplified (linear) chemical formula of a saturated fatty acid is shown in Figure 7.1. Observe that the carbon atom (tetravalent) binds chemically through four bonds (represented by lines in the formulas), the oxygen atom (bivalent) through two bonds, and the hydrogen atom (monovalent) through one bond. The chemical formula shown in Figure 7.1 can be represented in a more compact way as $H_3C(CH_2)_7COOH$, that is, a methyl radical (H_3C-) bonded to seven $-(CH_2)-$ groups and ending with a carboxyl radical ($-COOH$). Another example of a saturated fatty acid is the *stearic acid*, with 18 carbon atoms in its chain and having the chemical formula $H_3C(CH_2)_{16}COOH$. All saturated fatty acids have only single chemical bonds between the

> Saturated fatty acids have only single chemical bonds between the carbon atoms in their molecular chain.

carbon atoms in their molecular chain.

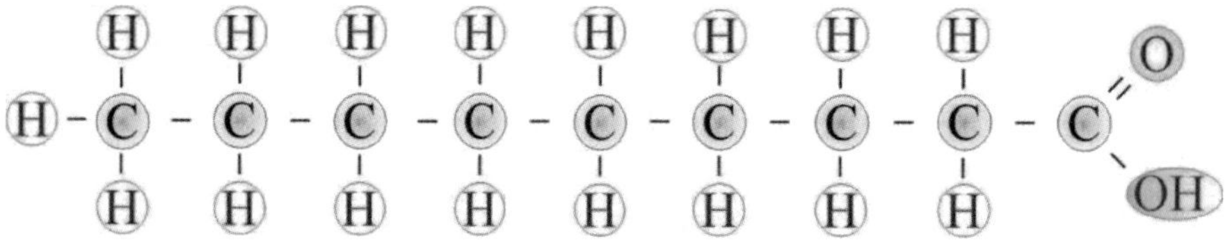

(Methyl) **(Carboxyl)**

FIGURE 7.1 – Simplified (linear) chemical formula of a saturated fatty acid. In this example, the molecule contains nine carbon atoms in its molecular chain.

Unsaturated fatty acids possess fewer hydrogen atoms than their saturated correspondents and can be monounsaturated (when they have only one double bond in their hydrocarbon chain) or polyunsaturated (when they have more than one double bond). The abbreviations UFA, MUFA, and PUFA, usually present in the labels of some industrialized foods, refer respectively to the expressions *Unsaturated Fatty Acid*, *MonoUnsaturated Fatty Acid*, and *PolyUnsaturated Fatty Acid*. One example of a MUFA is shown in Figure 7.2. Figure 7.3 shows the simplified (linear) chemical formula of a PUFA (diunsaturated, in this example).

Most of the oils from seeds and vegetables have medium chains of carbon atoms, while butter and animal fats have smaller carbon chains. The fish and marine oils are unique in the sense that they are constituted of long chains of carbon atoms.

Saturated fats are usually solid at ambient temperatures and are present mainly in foods from animal sources, with the exception of some saturated fats of vegetable origin, such as those present in tropical plants (e.g., coconut, heart of palm, and cacao). They are found in meats, poultry, eggs, milk, and milk derivatives such as cheese and yogurt. Monounsaturated and polyunsaturated fats occur generally in liquid form at room temperature (usually called oils) and are found in vegetable oils from nuts, seeds, and grains (e.g., corn, soy, canola, sunflower, olive, and peanuts). The natural fatty acids of the saturated, monounsaturated, and polyunsaturated types coexist in different relative proportions in practically all foods that contain fats.

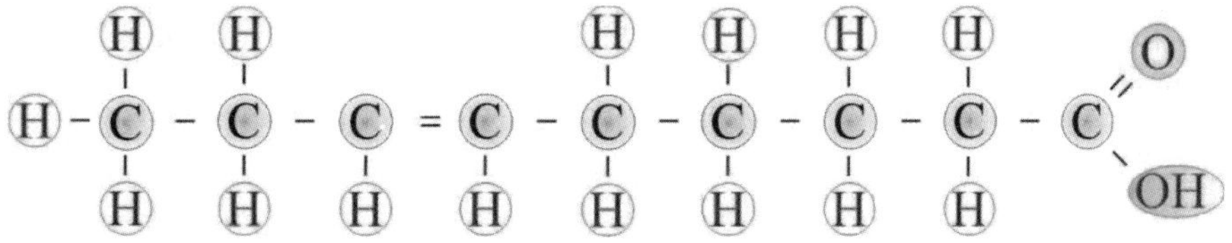

FIGURE 7.2 – Simplified (linear) chemical formula of a monounsaturated fatty acid (MUFA).

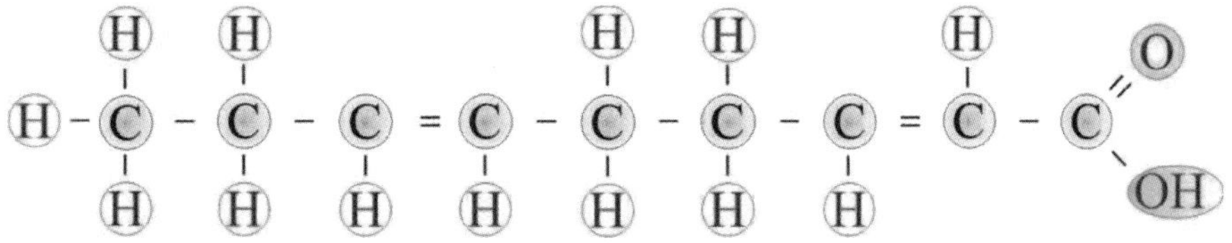

FIGURE 7.3 – Simplified (linear) chemical formula of a polyunsaturated fatty acid (PUFA). In this example, a diunsaturated fatty acid.

7.4 THE OMEGA NOMENCLATURE

In the *omega* (ω) nomenclature system used in organic chemistry, the carbon atoms in the fatty acid molecular chain are counted from the radical methyl (–CH$_3$). In chemistry, the chain terminal that contains the radical methyl is considered as the end of the fatty acid molecule and the carboxyl radical as the beginning. For example, the denomination omega-6, used in the description of some unsaturated fatty acids, means that the first double bond occurs in the sixth carbon atom counted from the methyl radical. In the examples shown in Figures 7.2 and 7.3, an omega-3 unsaturated fatty acid is shown. Although the body can convert some small-chain fatty acids into long-chain acids, the position of the first double bond remains, so omega-3 unsaturated fatty acids cannot be converted into omega-6.

Omega-3 fatty acids are found in fish oils, flaxseed, and, in smaller proportions, in egg yolk, nuts, and the seeds and leaves of many plants. Three important groups belong to the omega-3 family: *linolenic* or *alpha-linolenic acid* (LNA), *eicosapentaenoic acid* (EPA), and *docosahexaenoic acid* (DHA). The best sources of EPA and DHA are fish oils, but the body can produce these fatty acids starting from LNA and other nutrients. Flaxseeds constitute an excellent source of LNA.

The natural fatty acids of the saturated, monounsaturated, and polyunsaturated types coexist in different relative proportions in practically all foods that contain fats.

Omega-6 fatty acids are found in plant seeds and vegetable oils such as corn, soy, sunflower, and saffron. Three important groups are included in this family: linoleic acid (LA), gamma-linolenic acid (GLA), and arachidonic acid (AA). Normally, GLA is not a part of the diet of most people. It is found predominantly in primrose oil and the seeds of borage and gooseberry. GLA is important for the metabolism of prostaglandins and can be produced by the body starting from LA and other nutrients when these are present in the diet. GLA has 18 carbon atoms in its molecular chain, with three double bonds occurring each in the carbons 6, 9, and 12.

A third important group consists of the *omega-9 fatty acids*, represented by *oleic acid*, a monounsaturated fatty acid present in olive oil, macadamia, and, in smaller proportions, in avocado, peanuts, and nuts. Oleic acid has 18 carbon atoms in its molecular chain, with a double bond in the middle of the chain. Its chemical formula can be represented as $H_3C(CH_2)_7(CH)_2(CH_2)_7COOH$.

Table 7.1 shows a list of some oils and fats with their relative proportions, in percentage, of saturated and unsaturated fatty acids. Note that the best proportion of omega-3 to omega-6 fatty acids occurs in flaxseed oil, followed by canola oil. The best sources of monounsaturated fatty acids (MUFAs) are macadamia and olive oil, followed by canola, peanut, and sesame oils. Milk butter and coconut fat are rich in saturated fatty acids (SFAs), but all oils have some percentage of saturated fats.

TABLE 7.1 – Relative proportion (in percentage) of fatty acids present in some oils and fats (percentages relative to the fatty component only).

OIL OR FAT	SFA	MUFA	OMEGA-6	OMEGA-3
Canola	6	62	22	10
Coconut	92	6	2	0
Corn	13	25	61	1
Flaxseed	9	18	16	57
Macadamia	14	81	5	0
Milk butter	66	30	2	2
Olive oil	14	77	8	1
Peanut	18	49	33	0
Pecan	16	28	51	5
Saffron	10	13	77	0
Sesame	13	46	41	0
Soy	15	24	54	7
Sunflower	11	20	69	0

Note: The terms SFA and MUFA refer to saturated fatty acids and monounsaturated fatty acids, respectively.

7.5 THE DELTA NUMBERING SYSTEM

*A*nother numbering system used to identify the double bonds in the carbon atoms of the fatty acid molecular chain is called the *delta system*. In this system, the carbon atoms are counted from the carboxyl radical. In a simplified nomenclature, the system first specifies the number of carbon atoms in the molecular chain and the number of double bonds, separated by two points. The

Greek letter delta (Δ) follows with superscript numbers that specify the positions of the double bonds, counting the carbon atoms from the carboxyl radical. For example, GLA is designated as 18:3 $\Delta^{6,9,12}$, oleic acid as 18:1 Δ^9, and palmitic acid (saturated) as 16:0.

> In the omega system the double bonds in the chain of carbon atoms are counted from the methyl radical.

Table 7.2 shows a list of some of the main fatty acids present in human body tissues and their nomenclature. The relative composition in percentage of the fatty acids present in the fatty part of some foods is shown in Table 7.3.

7.6 CIS AND TRANS CONFIGURATIONS

*T*o complicate things, the double bonds between carbon atoms can occur in two different configurations: *cis* and *trans*. The molecules have a three-dimensional structure, and the chemical bonds project themselves spatially in different directions from the carbon atoms. When both hydrogen atoms involved in the double bond between carbon atoms appear in the same side, the configuration is called cis, and, when they are in opposite sides, the configuration is called trans, as shown in Figure 7.4. All naturally occurring fatty acids in mammals are of the cis configuration.

Chemical substances that have the same chemical formula but a different spatial arrangement are called *stereoisomers* (or *spatial isomers*). The trans fatty acids (artificial substances) react biochemically differently from the cis fatty acids (natural substances). The trans configuration makes the fatty acids more stable (less susceptible to oxidation) than the natural cis form. The trans fatty acids behave somewhat as saturated fats (more stable), even though they are unsaturated. The cis configuration is the form normally used by the body for the production of cell membranes and hormones. The trans fats incorporate differently in the

> In the *cis* configuration the hydrogen atoms appear in the same side, around a carbon-carbon double bond, whereas in the *trans* configuration they occur in opposite sides.

triglyceride and phospholipid molecules, when compared to the cis form, and they compromise body metabolism.

TABLE 7.2 – Some important fatty acids in human body tissues.

Descriptive name	Systematic name	Number of carbon atoms	Double bonds	Delta notation	Omega notation
Acetic		2	0	2:0	
Lauric	Dodecanoic	12	0	12:0	
Miristic	Tetradecanoic	14	0	14:0	
Palmitic	Hexadecanoic	16	0	16:0	
Palmitoleic	Hexadecenoic	16	1	$16:1\,\Delta^{9}$	$\omega-7$
Estearic	Octadecanoic	18	0	18:0	
Oleic	Octadecenoic	18	1	$18:1\,\Delta^{9}$	$\omega-9$
Linoleic	Octadecadienoic	18	2	$18:2\,\Delta^{9,12}$	$\omega-6$
Linolenic	Octadecatrienoic	18	3	$18:3\,\Delta^{9,12,15}$	$\omega-3$
Gamma-Linolenic	Eicosatrienoic	20	3	$20:3\,\Delta^{8,11,14}$	$\omega-6$
Arachidonic	Eicosatetraenoic	20	4	$20:4\,\Delta^{5,8,11,14}$	$\omega-6$
EPA	Eicosapentaenoic	20	5	$20:5\,\Delta^{5,8,11,14,17}$	$\omega-3$
DHA	Docosahexaenoic	22	6	$22:6\,\Delta^{4,7,10,13,16,19}$	$\omega-3$

Artificially made fats such as margarine and vegetable fats (solid at room temperature) undergo an industrial transformation process called *hydrogenation* that converts liquid vegetable oils into a form that is solid and stable at room temperature. These fats, in which some of the double bonds between carbon atoms (of unsaturated vegetable oils) are artificially saturated with hydrogen atoms, are called *partially hydrogenated vegetable fats*, and they have a great number of molecules in the trans configuration, generated in the industrial hydrogenation process. These artificial fats are antinutrients that interfere in a harmful way with fatty acid metabolism.

TABLE 7.3 – Relative composition (in percentage) of fatty acids present in the fatty part of some foods (percentages relative to the fatty component only).

FATTY ACID / FOOD	Lauric	Miristic	Palmitic	Palmitoleic	Estearic	Oleic	Linoleic	Others
Bacon		2	25	3	15	45	9	1
Beef tallow		3	26	3	25	36	2	5
Coconut oil	54	18	8		2	5	1	12
Corn oil			10		2	31	56	1
Cotton seed oil			20		2	18	60	
Milk butter	3	11	31	3	14	30	2	6
Olive oil			11		2	79	7	1
Safflower oil			5		2	17	76	
Soy oil			10		4	24	54	8

Note: Absence of a value means that the amount is less than 0.5 %.

7.7 BASIC CHARACTERISTICS OF FATTY ACIDS

*I*n summary, fatty acids are substances insoluble in water (soluble in fat), and each type has specific biochemical properties that depend on some basic chemical characteristics:

➢ The number of carbon atoms or carbon chain length.

➢ The number of double bonds in the carbon atom molecular chain.

➢ The position of the double bonds, specified by the omega (ω) or by the delta (Δ) numbering system.

➢ Whether or not the unsaturated fatty acid possesses the cis or trans configuration.

7.8 ESSENTIAL FATTY ACIDS

*T*hree fatty acids that are necessary to our health are not synthesized by the body: *linoleic acid* (LA), *linolenic acid* (LNA), and *arachidonic acid* (AA). These polyunsaturated fatty acids must be provided by the diet and, for this reason, they are called *essential*. The other fatty acids, necessary for good health, can be synthesized by the body starting from carbohydrates, proteins, and fats present in food, together with some vitanutrients. Essential fatty acids are necessary for normal growth, brain function, and for health of nerves, arteries, and blood.

CIS Configuration   **TRANS Configuration**

FIGURE 7.4 – The spatial orientation of hydrogen atoms in the configuration of the stereoisomers *cis* and *trans*, around a carbon-carbon double bond in unsaturated fatty acids.

Linoleic acid (LA) belongs to the omega-6 family and is found in the seeds of plants and their oils, such as corn, soy, and sunflower. It consists of a molecular chain with 18 carbon atoms, having two double bonds that each occur in the carbon atoms 6 and 9, counted from the methyl radical. Its simplified chemical formula is shown in Figure 7.5, where each vertex of the sawed line represents a carbon atom (the hydrogen atoms are not shown in this illustration). LA can also be represented as $18:2\ \Delta^{9,12}$.

Essential fatty acids are fundamental for our health and cannot be synthesized by the body. They must be obtained from the alimentary diet.

Linolenic or *alpha-linolenic acid* (LNA) belongs to the omega-3 family of unsaturated fatty acids and is found in fish and flaxseed oils. It consists of a molecular chain with 18 carbon atoms, with three double bonds that each occur in the carbon atoms 3, 6, and 9, counted from the methyl radical, as shown in Figure 7.6. LNA may also be represented as 18:3 $\Delta^{9,12,15}$.

Arachidonic acid (AA) is a polyunsaturated fatty acid that belongs to the omega-6 family and is found in meats and cheese. It consists of a molecular chain with 20 carbon atoms and four double bonds that each occur in the carbon atoms 6, 9, 12, and 15, counted from the methyl radical. Its simplified chemical formula is shown in Figure 7.7. AA may also be represented as 20:4 $\Delta^{5,8,11,14}$. However, AA may be synthesized from LA, when present in the diet, and may not be considered essential in some cases.

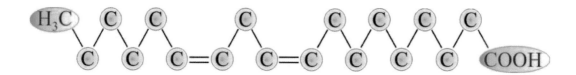

FIGURE 7.5 – Schematic formula of the essential linoleic acid (LA). It belongs to the omega-6 family and can also be represented as 18:2 $\Delta^{9,12}$. Hydrogen atoms of the fatty acid molecular chain are not shown.

For good health, it is important that the fatty acids of both omega-3 and omega-6 families be consumed together in similar proportions, because a proper balance between them is fundamental for the metabolism of prostaglandins. The best proportion of omega-3 to omega-6 is found in flaxseed oil, followed by canola oil (refer to Table 7.1).

The functions of essential fatty acids, also known as EFAs, include the regulation of cholesterol metabolism, the maintenance of the integrity and functional regulation of all cellular membranes (constituted mainly of fats), and the production of prostaglandins, which are active substances similar to hormones (chemical messengers), but of short duration and reach, that regulate almost all body functions. The trans fatty acids, produced in the partial hydrogenation of vegetable oils and which are added to a variety of industrial foods, impair the use of EFAs by the body. The presence of trans-LA blocks the utilization of cis-LA (and the production of GLA), increasing the amount of EFAs needed by the body and aggravating the symptoms of EFA deficiency.

The deficiency of EFAs impairs brain function and may lead to a reduction in the amount and size of brain cells, as well as lack of communication between them, which may cause thinking, learning, and growth problems. Current evidence indicates that LA and GLA have a protective effect against *atherosclerosis* (narrowing and hardening of the arteries) and cancer.

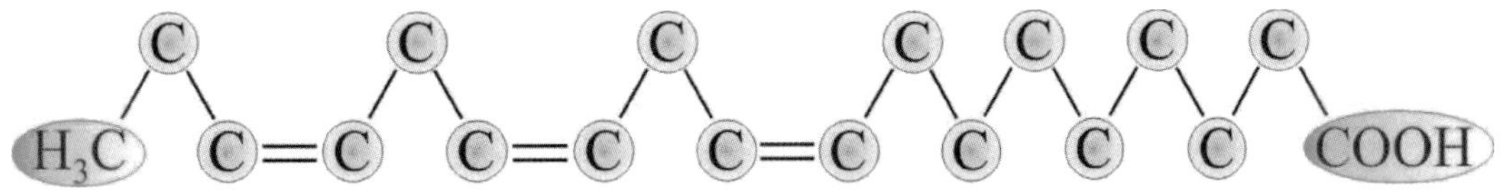

FIGURE 7.6 – Schematic formula of the essential linolenic acid (LNA). It belongs to the omega-3 family and can also be represented as 18:3 $\Delta^{9,12,15}$. Hydrogen atoms of the fatty acid molecular chain are not shown.

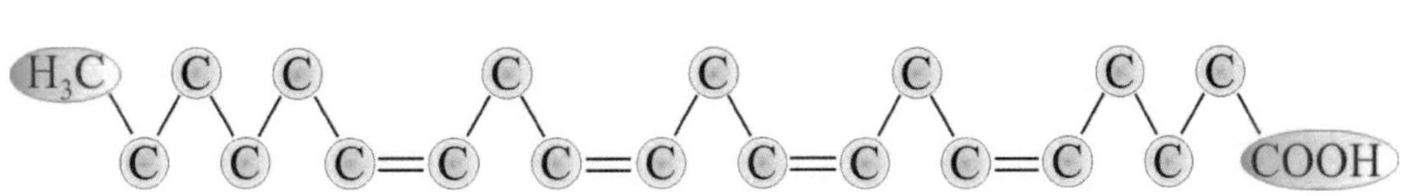

FIGURE 7.7 – Schematic formula of the essential arachidonic acid (AA). It belongs to the omega-6 family and can also be represented as 20:4 $\Delta^{5,8,11,14}$. Hydrogen atoms of the fatty acid molecular chain are not shown.

7.9 TRIGLYCERIDES

The fat stored in the body, as well as most of the fat present in foods, is constituted of *triglycerides*. This type of lipid receives this name because it is formed of three fatty acid molecular chains linked to a *glycerol* molecule. They are also called *triacylglycerols*. The glycerol molecule, which chemically belongs to the organic alcohol family, consists of a chain of three carbon atoms, having a hydroxyl radical (–OH) bonded to each carbon atom, as shown in Figure 7.8.

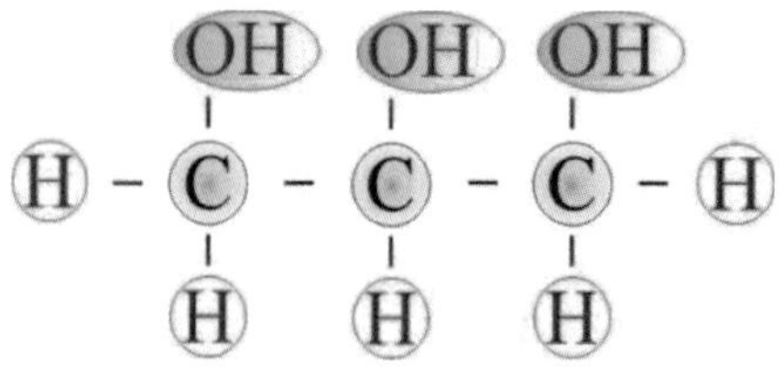

FIGURE 7.8 – Chemical formula of the glycerol molecule. This substance belongs to the organic family of alcohols.

> Triglycerides are constituted of three fatty acid molecules linked to a glycerol molecule.

An example of a lipid representative of the triglycerides is the *tripalmitate glycerol*, whose chemical formula is shown in Figure 7.9. This lipid constitutes a saturated fat, because all carbon atoms in the component fatty acid chains (*palmitic acid*) are linked through single bonds. Other saturated fats have a larger or smaller number of chemical groups ($-CH_2-$). The triglycerides may also be constituted of unsaturated fatty acids.

> The glycerol molecule belongs to the organic alcohol family and has three carbon atoms each bonded to a hydroxyl (–OH) radical.

During digestion, the triglycerides from food are broken down by pancreatic enzymes almost completely into glycerol and the component fatty acid molecules. However, as a result of incomplete digestion, some monoglycerides and diglycerides may also be formed. The glycerol, the free fatty acids, the diglycerides, and the monoglycerides are absorbed in the bloodstream with the help of bile salts (for emulsification). These lipids are subsequently rebuilt by the liver into triglycerides that circulate in the bloodstream through *lipoproteins*. They are used for energy production, prostaglandin synthesis, and other functions, or they are stored in body fat tissues for later use.

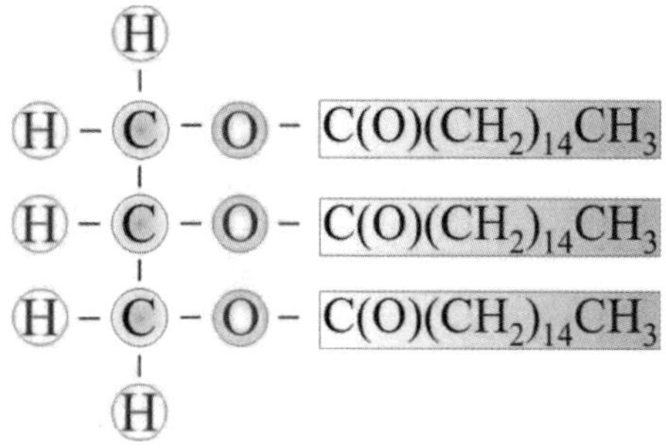

$$
\begin{array}{c}
\text{H} \\
| \\
\text{H} - \text{C} - \text{O} - \boxed{\text{C(O)(CH}_2)_{14}\text{CH}_3} \\
| \\
\text{H} - \text{C} - \text{O} - \boxed{\text{C(O)(CH}_2)_{14}\text{CH}_3} \\
| \\
\text{H} - \text{C} - \text{O} - \boxed{\text{C(O)(CH}_2)_{14}\text{CH}_3} \\
| \\
\text{H}
\end{array}
$$

FIGURE 7.9 – Chemical formula of the tripalmitate glycerol, a triglyceride.

As described in the chapter on carbohydrates, excess of sugars and starches resulting from eating too many carbohydrates may be converted by the liver into triglycerides, which can be stored as body fat. High blood levels of triglycerides are associated with a greater risk of developing cardiovascular disease.

7.10 PHOSPHOLIPIDS

*P*hospholipids constitute a class of lipids that have the phosphorus mineral in their molecule. Similarly to triglycerides, they are structured in the glycerol molecule. The most well-known members of this class are *lecithin* (phosphatidyl-choline) and *choline*. Lecithin has two fatty acid molecules bonded to a glycerol molecule, while choline has three. These lipids constitute a great part of the cellular membranes and are fundamental to life. Lecithin, also called *phosphatidyl-choline*, can be synthesized by the liver and is not an essential fat.

The phospholipids have both hydrophilic (soluble in water) and hydrophobic (insoluble in water) parts that make them good emulsifiers. Lecithin is a natural emulsifier of fats, and it can liquefy fat present in the blood vessels

> Phospholipids possess the phosphorus mineral in their molecule and are also structured in the glycerol molecule.

and prevent the formation of plaque on arterial walls. Studies have shown that lecithin helps to diminish excessive levels of cholesterol in many individuals. It is an essential element of all body cells and acts to protect the nervous system cells. It also serves as a primary source of choline, a precursor of *acetyl-choline*, one of the most valuables neurotransmitters. The properties of lecithin and choline are discussed in more detail in another chapter.

7.11 STEROLS

Sterols are constituted of large and complex molecules that involve carbon atom chains that are interconnected and closed in the form of rings. The most well-known lipid belonging to this class is *cholesterol*, but vitamin D, the sexual hormone *testosterone*, and bile acids also belong to this class.

> Cholesterol, vitamin D, testosterone, and bile acids are members of the sterol family.

Cholesterol is present in all tissues of the human body and in animals, mainly in the liver, and possesses important biochemical properties. It is soluble in oils and fats but is not found in vegetables. Its chemical formula ($C_{27}H_{45}OH$) involves various carbon atom chains closed in the form of rings. It constitutes the raw material to make hormones, vitamin D, and cell membranes, and it is fundamental for good health. Cholesterol is a normal component of the brain, spinal cord, nervous system, liver, and blood. Cholesterol is vitally important for brain function and 25% of the cholesterol in the body is found in the brain, where it plays important roles. Low cholesterol is associated with an increased risk for depression and even death. The many properties of cholesterol and its body metabolism are considered in other chapters.

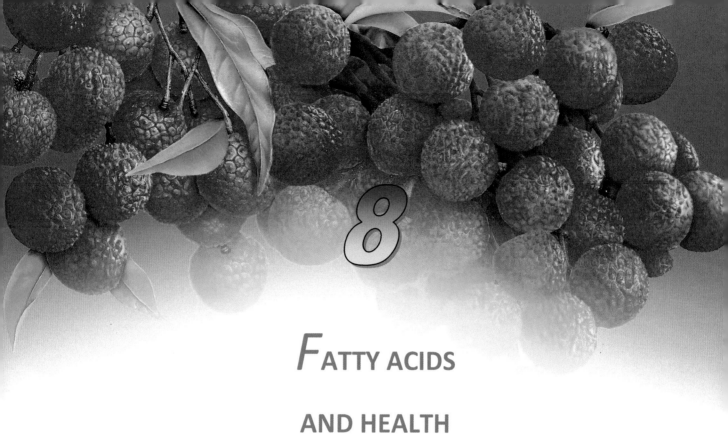

*F*ATTY ACIDS

AND HEALTH

8.1 PROSTAGLANDINS

*P*rostaglandins (PGs) and *eicosanoids* are substances similar to hormones (chemical messengers), but of short duration and reach, that regulate all the organs and cells, affecting our health in many forms. Unlike hormones, PGs are not transported through the bloodstream to a remote location in the body, but they act in the vicinity of the cells that produce them. Most PGs are decomposed in seconds or minutes, so their effects are limited to neighboring tissues. These substances control a large number of essential body functions and are involved in a variety of processes such as blood coagulation, arterial pressure regulation, cardiovascular disorders, inflammation control, pain and fever occurrence, hormone production, arthritis, premenstrual stress, colic, headaches, allergic reactions, asthma, swelling, fertility and reproduction, glaucoma, and perhaps cancer.

PGs cannot be obtained through food, because they are constituted of complex molecules that are destroyed by the digestive process. The body does not store PGs, and they are produced in each body tissue, according to our momentary need, starting from some fatty acids. Their effect is of short duration, because they are rapidly deactivated by enzymes. The functional integrity of many organ systems depends on a balance or equilibrium between different PGs that act in opposite ways or in antagonism.

8.2 PROSTAGLANDIN FUNCTIONS

The body functions of a great number of PGs are already well known. Of these, the ones that belong to the groups designated as the *E family* and the *F family* seem to be the most important. They are represented in a compact form as the PGE and the PGF families. Another PG family of particular interest is the *I family*, of which *prostacyclin* (PGI_2) is a particularly potent cell regulator. Prostacyclin is synthesized from arachidonic acid (AA) and is the main PG produced by the vascular *endothelium*, acting as vasodilator (particularly for the coronary arteries) and as a blood anticlotting agent, preventing blood platelet aggregation and adherence to the endothelium surface. *Thromboxane* A_2 (TXA_2), also synthesized from AA, is the main PG produced by blood platelets (blood cells that have the form of small plates, half the size of red cells, involved in blood clotting) and it produces effects opposite to those of prostacyclin, because it contracts the arteries and starts blood platelet aggregation. Its activity is of short duration with a half-life of about 30 seconds.

In the PGE family, the most important members are PGE_1 and PGE_3. The tissue levels of PGE_1 are of crucial importance for overall health. A decrease in PGE_1 levels leads to a potentially catastrophic series of problems that include enhanced vascular reactivity, enhanced tendency for blood coagulation, elevated cholesterol production, diabetic propensity for insulin secretion, enhanced risk for autoimmune diseases, inflammatory disorders, and susceptibility

> Prostaglandins (PGs) are substances similar to hormones, but of short reach and duration, that regulate all body organs and cells.

to depression. PGE_1 is necessary for normal functioning of the *T-cells* (the cells that reject foreign invaders) of the immune system. It also reduces the formation of inflammation-producing PGE_2 by blocking AA release from storage and prevents arthritis.

The subscript numbers in the PG notation refer to the type of fatty acid that is used as a starting point for PG synthesis. The subscript number 1 is used to denote the PG series produced from *gamma-linolenic acid* (GLA), which belongs to the omega-6 unsaturated fatty acids (not omega-3, as the name may suggest) and is found in primrose and borage oils. GLA can also be synthesized by the body starting from the essential *cis-linoleic acid* (cis-LA) and some vitanutrients, as shown in Figure 8.1.

The conversion of cis-LA into GLA depends on a specific enzyme known as *delta-6-desaturase* (D6D), which is produced with the help of vitamins C, B_3, and B_6 and the minerals zinc and magnesium. However, some blocking factors can interfere with this synthesis such as the presence of trans fats, excess saturated fats, cholesterol, and alcohol, the presence of radiation and carcinogenic substances,

> The numerical subscripts in the prostaglandin notation refer to the type of fatty acid that is used as a starting point for prostaglandin synthesis.

advanced age, deficiency of vitamins B_3, B_6, and C, and deficiency of minerals such as zinc and magnesium. When GLA synthesis from cis-LA is blocked, it may be necessary to get GLA from the diet in order to help the body produce optimum amounts of PGs.

The subscript number 2 denotes the PG series produced from *arachidonic acid* (AA), an essential unsaturated omega-6 fatty acid found in fats from animal origin (e.g., meats and cheeses). The *eicosanoids* are derived from AA, and their name comes from the fact that this polyunsaturated omega-6 fatty acid has 20 carbon atoms in its molecular chain (from the Greek *eikosi*, which means *twenty*). Related compounds include prostacyclins, thromboxanes, and leucotrienes.

The subscript number 3 denotes the PG series that are synthesized from the fatty acids *eicosapentaenoic* (EPA) and *docosahexaenoic* (DHA), which belong to the unsaturated omega-3 family, found in fish oils.

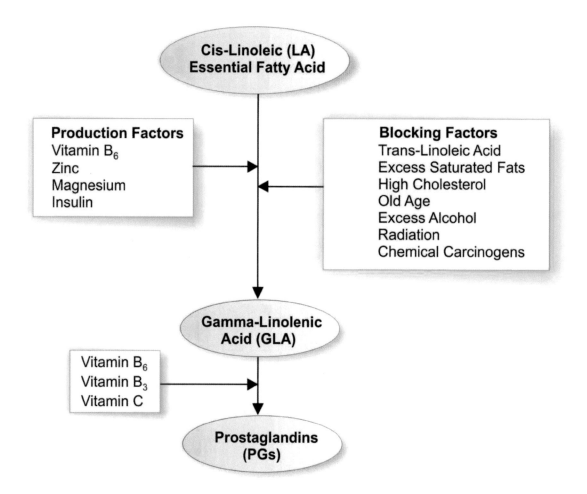

FIGURE 8.1 - Nutrients necessary for the conversion of essential cis-linolenic acid (cis-LA) into gamma-linolenic acid (GLA) and blocking factors that interfere with this synthesis.

The PGs synthesized from GLA (subscript 1) and EPA and DHA (subscript 3) perform desirable functions that are sometimes neutralized by some PGs produced from AA (subscript 2). PGE_1 and PGE_3 protect against heart attacks caused by blood clotting. PGE_1, PGE_3, and PGI_2 prevent blood platelets from becoming sticky, with tendency for clotting, but PGE_2 promotes platelet aggregation, which is the first step for blood coagulation. A proper balance between them maintains adequate blood coagulation. PGE_1 also exerts a diuretic action, whereas PGE_2 promotes salt retention by the kidneys, increasing water retention in the body. Consequently, PGE_2 is a potential factor related to high blood pressure. Current evidence shows that GLA and its derivative PGE_1, as well as PGE_3, have anti-inflammatory properties, making them excellent healing agents, whereas AA and its derivative PGE_2 have inflammatory properties.

Nevertheless, AA does not always have undesirable characteristics. It is the most abundant fatty acid in the brain and is fundamental for healthy functioning of this organ. Health problems may arise only when AA is present in excess or when it is not properly balanced with adequate amounts of GLA, EPA, and DHA.

Aspirin (the popular name for *acetylsalicylic acid*), an analgesic, antipyretic, and anti-inflammatory agent, normally used to alleviate pain, fever, and inflammation, acts in the body inhibiting the synthesis of prostacyclins, thromboxanes, and prostaglandins produced from AA (precursor). The *leucotrienes*, also synthesized from AA, are insensitive to aspirin and are associated with inflammatory and hypersensitivity disturbances such as asthma. Aspirin is also commonly used as an anti-inflammatory agent for the cardiovascular system.

In summary, an adequate balance between fatty acids in the diet and appropriate ingestion of EFAs is fundamental for the maintenance of a healthy equilibrium between the PGs. Unfortunately, many people consume too much AA and trans-LA, and very small quantities of GLA, cis-LA, EPA, and DHA. Many researchers affirm that various diseases arise as the result of an imbalance between the PGs.

8.3 BROWN FAT TISSUE AND THERMOGENESIS

*B*rown fat tissue (or simply *brown fat*) refers to a unique type of fat that differs from the normal fat deposits (or *white fat*) stored in the body for eventual use as an energy source. The name can be misleading, because brown fat has the property to generate thermal energy by burning elementary food constituents, as compared to white fat, which is an energetic deposit to be burned. Its brownish color is caused by the high concentration of *mitochondria*, the tiny cellular units that act as power plants for energy production, allowing brown fat to burn the elementary metabolic fuels from excess calories.

Brown fat surrounds vital organs such as the heart, kidneys, adrenal glands, and the main blood vessels of the thorax. This tissue is also found in the posterior region of the neck, and along the spinal column. Two functions of brown fat are adaptation to cold climates and control of body weight.

The complex processes of brown fat may explain why some people expend more calories than others and remain slim, even while ingesting excess food calories, and others easily gain weight (their excess food calories are stored as body fat).

The brown fat tissue generates thermal energy (calories) for body heat, not energy for body movement (work), in a process called *thermogenesis* (*thermo* means *heat*, and *genesis* means *creation*). Although brown fat constitutes only about 10% or less of total body fat, it is responsible for about 25% of all calories expended by all tissues combined.

Obese people who have a tendency to store excess food calories as body fat probably have insufficient amounts of brown fat tissue or an inefficient mechanism for activating thermogenesis in these tissues.

An adequate balance between fatty acids in the diet is fundamental for the maintenance of a healthy equilibrium between the PGs.

Research has demonstrated that the addition of essential fatty acids (EFAs) and gamma-linolenic acid (GLA) to the diet is fundamental to increase the metabolic rate and to activate brown fat thermogenesis. GLA acts as a precursor of some prostaglandins that activate the fat-burning process in the brown fat mitochondria, being notably efficient in reducing body fat and in weight loss.

8.4 HYDROGENATED VEGETABLE OILS: FROM GOOD TO BAD

*H*ydrogenation of unsaturated vegetable oils is the most common way to transform healthy natural oils into artificial fat products that can cause serious health issues. This is done by the food industry on a large scale for commercial profit, and relatively cheap vegetable oils (liquid at normal room temperature) are transformed into margarine (solid at room temperature and more stable). Margarine is used in a variety of industrially prepared foods, such as cookies, salty snacks, biscuits, spaghetti, frozen foods, and other products that have a long lifespan on supermarket shelves.

In hydrogenation, a process that uses pressure and metallic catalysts such as nickel and aluminum, hydrogen atoms are added into the double bonds of the molecular chain of unsaturated vegetable oils. In the molecules where all double bonds are saturated with

> The addition of EFAs and GLA to the diet is fundamental to increase the metabolic rate and to activate brown fat thermogenesis.

hydrogen, a saturated fat is produced. Partial hydrogenation results in molecules with double bonds between the carbon atoms in the molecular chain, or unsaturated artificial fat molecules, that may have cis or trans configurations. Hydrogenation also produces fragments of artificial fatty acids and other modified molecules that may be toxic. Some studies associate the mineral aluminum, used as a catalyst, to the Alzheimer's disease (mental senility) in old age. While the body can produce cell membranes and hormones from the cis form, the fatty acids in the trans configuration interfere with the normal processing of natural fatty acids in the body.

> The trans fats affect negatively the metabolism of essential fatty acids and block the development of prostaglandins.

Current research shows that the trans fatty

acids are *antinutrients* that aggressively interfere with body biochemistry. Although what happens with the trans isomer in the body is not known exactly, countless studies have consistently shown that the trans fats increase blood levels of the *low-density lipoprotein* (LDL), popularly known as bad cholesterol, decrease blood levels of the *high-density lipoprotein* (HDL), popularly known as good cholesterol, and interfere with the liver's detoxification system. They also increase the blood levels of triglycerides and of a substance known as lipoprotein-(*a*), both of which are linked to cardiovascular diseases.

The trans fats negatively affect the metabolism of essential fatty acids and block the development of prostaglandins, which regulate the cardiovascular system, reproductive system, central nervous system, and immune system. Many diseases result from an imbalance in the prostaglandins. Research continues to show that hydrogenated vegetable oils in the trans configuration make blood platelets (responsible for the blood coagulation mechanism) more sticky than normal, thereby increasing the tendency for clot formation in vessels and promoting cardiovascular diseases and arterial obstructions in the heart, brain, and other parts of the body. Many researchers affirm that the trans fats (not saturated fats) constitute the food link for high blood cholesterol and cardiac disease.

> The food industry uses hydrogenated vegetable oils (vegetable fats), with trans fats, in many supermarket food products.

Currently, the margarine industry has diminished the amount of trans fats in this type of industrialized product. However, the food industry continues to use hydrogenated vegetable oils (with trans fats) in many food products, such as biscuits, cookies, potato chips, ice creams, frozen foods, and other supermarket products. It is advisable to read the labels of industrialized products to select foods with no trans fats and without hydrogenated vegetable oils or vegetable fats. Some food labels may read "no trans fats" even though they contain hydrogenated vegetable oils or vegetable fats, because the label information considers as absence of trans fats when the amount present is below a certain limit, per some grams of food, and not an absolute zero.

8.5 SATURATED FATS: THE SCAPEGOAT

Saturated fats and proteins from animal food sources such as meat, poultry, fish, eggs, milk, and milk derivatives have been part of the human diet for thousands of years. However, in the last few decades, saturated fats have been associated with higher blood cholesterol levels and the risk of cardiovascular disease. Fearing foods that contain animal fat and cholesterol, many people have eliminated from their diet good sources of complete proteins from animal origin, including eggs and milk derivatives, and used margarine (artificial antinutrients) as a substitute for milk butter.

Evidence accumulated in the last century has shown that the increase in the incidence of cardiovascular diseases coincides with the increase in the consumption of sugars and refined foods that are rich in simple carbohydrates of high *glycemic index* (GI) and deprived of important nutrients, as well as of artificially hydrogenated vegetable oils. These substances were only recently introduced into the human diet. They are novelties to our body and interfere, in a harmful way, with body metabolism. Reduced consumption of foods rich in complete proteins and organic vegetables in general, and increased consumption of sugars and refined industrialized foods, has caused an increase in obesity, diabetes, and cardiovascular disease.

At the beginning of the 20th century, when animal fat constituted about 80% of total fat ingested, coronary and heart diseases were rare. According to specialists, there has been no research or clinical studies that demonstrate, in a *conclusive way*, an association between normal consumption of saturated fats (from animal or tropical foods) and the occurrence of cardiovascular disease.

It is believed that the potential dangers of saturated fat consumption were overestimated. Current evidence indicates that the lipids potentially dangerous to our health include: (1) artificial trans fats in margarine and in many industrialized food products that contain hydrogenated vegetable oils or vegetable fats; (2) refined polyunsaturated vegetable oils that are deprived of important nutrients and protecting antioxidant substances, such as the easily oxidized refined oils of soy, corn, sunflower, and saffron; and (3) oils heated to high temperatures for long periods, such as in fried foods, which deliver a cascade of *free radicals* (oxidizing substances) in the bloodstream that damage arteries and promote diseases.

Saturated fats constitute a fundamental part of the body metabolism, and if they are not ingested, the body produces them. Curiously, fats synthesized in the liver occur in the saturated form (saturated fat is not intrinsically harmful).

Due to genetic individuality, people respond differently to saturated fats. Their consumption may potentially be harmful only when consumed excessively and as part of an unbalanced diet that is deficient in nutrients and antioxidants (substances that neutralize free radicals), excessive in calories, full of sugar and refined *glycemic carbohydrates* (which impair metabolism of saturated fats), and when altered by oxidizing substances and free radicals generated by the metabolism and by toxins in food and the environment.

> There are no clinical studies or research that demonstrate, in a conclusive way, an association between normal consumption of saturated fats and the occurrence of cardiovascular disease.

Many clinical studies have demonstrated that saturated fats (animal and tropical) contain important fat-soluble vitamins and help in the absorption of these nutrients, as well as of *carotenoids*, antioxidants, minerals, and other nutrients in food. Many studies have shown that saturated fats protect against infection, aid some hormonal functions and bone growth, and protect the liver from foreign elements. When consumed in moderation, as part of a balanced diet that contains food rich in complete proteins, vitamins, minerals, essential fatty acids, and soluble fibers, saturated fats contribute to a healthy metabolism.

8.6 DAILY NEED FOR FATS

*T*he present recommendation is that no more than 30% of the calories ingested daily should come from fats. The quality or type of fat is more important, because a proper balance between the many different types of lipids is fundamental for good health. As a general rule, saturated fats such as those in meats, poultry, eggs, cheeses, milk, and milk derivatives should constitute about 10% of ingested calories. Monounsaturated fats of the omega-9 family such as those in olive oil, macadamias, avocados, nuts, and peanuts should total another 10%. The remaining 10% should come from non-oxidized polyunsaturated fats, with a good balance between fats of the omega-3 family (fish and flaxseeds) and of the omega-6 family, and including the essential fatty acids linoleic (LA), linolenic (LNA), and arachidonic (AA).

> About 30% of the daily ingested calories should come from fats, selected in such a way as to include the fatty acids necessary for good health.

People tend to ingest a large amount of omega-6 oils (sometimes, oxidized) and not enough omega-3 oils, and this imbalance may be harmful to their health. It is recommended to avoid refined vegetable oils that are easily oxidized, such as soy, corn, sunflower, and saffron oils. When heated to high temperatures (as in fried foods), these delicate refined oils become highly toxic substances that send a cascade of free radicals (such as lipid peroxides) into the bloodstream. Canola and peanut oils, as well as extra virgin olive oil, are more resistant to oxidation and capable of supporting more elevated temperatures without undergoing considerable transformation. As a general rule, fried foods should be avoided.

Nutritional researchers also recommend avoiding artificial vegetable fats (hydrogenated vegetable oils) that contain trans fats, which are present in many industrialized and frozen foods. A common misconception is that margarine is better than milk butter because it does not contain cholesterol. Before choosing between margarine or butter, consider other options, such as a light cheese or a creamy cheese (in which the fat is associated with good-quality protein and other nutrients), extra virgin olive oil, or peanut butter without sugar.

Foods that contain fats, including nuts and seeds, should be stored in opaque or dark canisters (away from direct light) and in a refrigerator to avoid oxidation.

Table 8.1 shows the relative composition of macronutrients (carbohydrates, proteins, and lipids) and calories in some foods rich in oils and fats. Tables showing the nutritional composition of a large number of foods are available at the website of the US Department of Agriculture (USDA) *http://www.ars.usda.gov/ba/bhnrc/ndl.*

TABLE 8.1 – Calories and relative composition of macronutrients (in grams) contained in some fat-rich foods.

FOOD (100g)	Cal	Carb	Prot	Fat	Sat	Unsat
Almonds	595	25	16	52	5	45
Brazil nuts	690	13	15	65	17	48
Cashew nuts	580	32	16	47	9	36
Flax seeds	390	27	19	23	3	19
Hazel nuts	640	14	20	61	4.5	54
Macadamias	710	14	8.5	74	11	60
Peanuts	585	21	24	50	7	40
Pecans	680	18	8	68	5.5	59
Pistachios	585	25	21	49	6	40
Pumpkin seeds	550	20	25	46	9	36
Sesame seeds	575	25	17	49	7	39
Sunflower seeds	580	18	23	50	5.5	43

Note: **Cal** = Calorie; **Carb** = Carbohydrate; **Prot** = Protein; **Fat** = Total fat;
       Sat = Saturated fat; **Unsat** = Unsaturated fat.

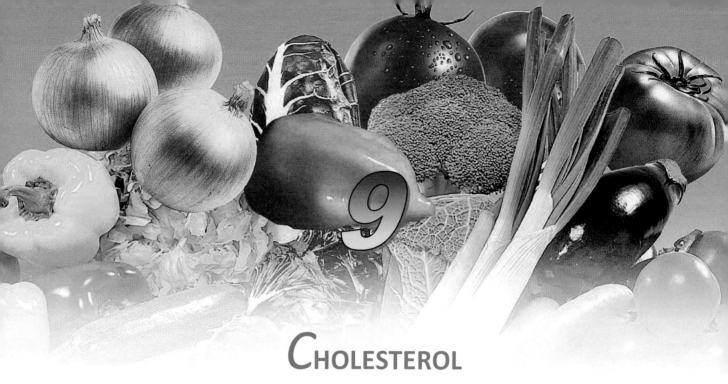

CHOLESTEROL

AND LIPOPROTEINS

9.1 THE IMPORTANCE OF CHOLESTEROL

*C*holesterol is the main *sterol* in the human body and is essential to life. Being a normal component of almost all tissues in the body, it is fundamental for good health and for sexual function, especially functions within the brain, spinal cord, nervous system, liver, and blood (*plasmatic lipoproteins*). Cholesterol is necessary for the production of cell membranes, the layers that surround nerves (*myelin sheath*), and the vital connections between the nerve cells in the brain (*synapses*). It is also an essential raw material for the synthesis of vitamin D, steroid hormones (including sex hormones), and bile acids. Although each person processes cholesterol properly for the most part, more than 90% of the cholesterol in the bloodstream ends up in the cells, where it carries out vital metabolic and structural functions.

The chemical formula of cholesterol is $C_{27}H_{45}OH$, and its molecular structure includes several closed chains of carbon atoms in the form of rings, as shown in Figure 9.1. In the figure, each vertex contains one of the carbon atoms, attached to one another, and to hydrogen atoms (omitted in the figure). In terms of chemical bonds, recall that carbon is tetravalent, oxygen is bivalent, and hydrogen is monovalent.

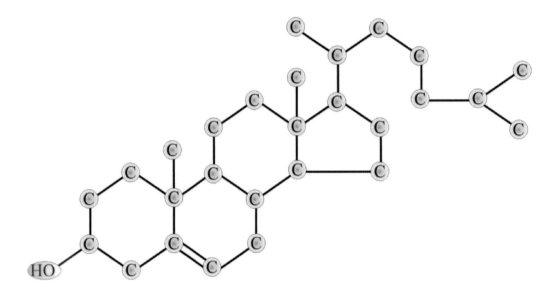

FIGURE 9.1 - Chemical formula of cholesterol ($C_{27}H_{45}OH$). Each vertex represents a carbon atom, attached to one another and to hydrogen atoms (not shown here).

Cholesterol occurs only in foods of animal origin and is not an essential fatty acid. (An essential fatty acid is one that the body cannot synthesize even though it is necessary for good health, so it must to be obtained from food.) It is so vital that almost all cells in the body, except neurons, can produce cholesterol, and one of the key functions of the liver is to synthesize cholesterol, as we usually do not get sufficient amounts from food. It is very important during early growth and development. We may say that an egg yolk is full of cholesterol because it takes a lot of cholesterol to build a healthy chicken, in the same way that it takes a lot of cholesterol to build and maintain a healthy human being.

Our liver produces about 2.5g to 3.5g of cholesterol each day, mainly from carbohydrates and fats to complement the amount captured from food. The liver also provides a complex system for transporting cholesterol and lipids in the bloodstream (lipoproteins), to move these substances around the body. Part of the cholesterol in the bloodstream is transformed into some hormones, part converts into vitamin D (from sunlight on our skin), part acts in the digestion and absorption of fats from food (in the form of bile, secreted by the liver for fat emulsification), and part is used for cellular structure maintenance.

It is believed that the fraction of cholesterol that is not used, when present in excess in the bloodstream, may be potentially harmful, especially if it contains oxidized cholesterol. Current evidence indicates that anomalies in the metabolism of cholesterol, or in its transport through the blood, may eventually cause the development of atherosclerosis. Some types of lipoproteins (the carriers of cholesterol in the bloodstream) are used as predictors of the risk of cardiovascular disease.

Many researchers and authors consider the *lipid hypothesis*, which asserts that saturated fat consumption and high blood levels of cholesterol cause atherosclerosis and coronary heart disease, to be erroneous or a harmful misconception. Massive volumes of scientific literature and clinical research indicate that heart disease is not caused simply by elevated blood cholesterol levels or by saturated fat consumption. The lipid hypothesis, by itself, seems to be scientifically invalid and must be seen under a much broader perspective, re-evaluated, or discarded.

It is usually accepted that the consumption of saturated fats raises blood cholesterol levels, but of the numerous controlled clinical trials examining dietary interventions for preventing heart disease, none has demonstrated a beneficial effect from saturated fat restriction. Numerous populations that consume high amounts of saturated fat have been observed to enjoy good health and extremely low rates of heart disease. There are

> Cholesterol is fundamental for good health and our liver produces about 2.5g to 3.5g each day, mainly from carbohydrates and fats.

many clinical studies contradicting the idea that saturated fat consumption, or high blood cholesterol levels, will cause heart disease. Still, controversy about this subject remains.

On the other hand, a low cholesterol level may cause health problems including anemia, excessive thyroid function, immune system deficiencies, infections, autoimmune disorders, and transient amnesia. In pregnant woman, a very low cholesterol level may cause childbirth defects.

Cholesterol is not an undesirable, or alien, chemical that must be removed from the diet, as some people may believe.

9.2 SERUM CHOLESTEROL LEVELS

*T*he amount of cholesterol in the bloodstream is determined by a combination of the following factors:

➢ The rate at which it is synthesized in the liver.

➢ The rate at which it is absorbed from food.

➢ The rate at which it is converted into bile acids and eliminated in the intestines.

➢ The rate at which the bile acids are reabsorbed in the small intestine and reconverted into cholesterol.

A dynamic steady state is continuously established between the loss rate (conversion into bile acids) and the other three rates. This dynamic steady state changes when these rates are altered, and they can be influenced by the nature of our food, by genetics, and by other factors. Cholesterol blood levels ranging from 160mg/l to about 230mg/l are considered normal.

Most of the cholesterol in the body is biosynthesized and does not originate from food cholesterol. Only about 20% to 30% of serum cholesterol comes from the cholesterol in food. However, it is well known that the liver acts in a compensatory way, producing more cholesterol when the amount from food decreases. Since 1970, from the large-scale and long-duration study conducted on the residents of Framingham, Massachusetts, which was designed to explore the correlating risk factors in the development of heart disease, it became evident that for the majority of people, restricting food cholesterol does not have a significant effect on the level of serum cholesterol, as the liver has a regenerative mechanism that reduces the rate of cholesterol synthesis when ingestion is increased and vice versa. Although most people have this feedback mechanism (balancing the amount obtained from food with the amounts synthesized in the liver and absorbed from the intestine), some people may have a less-efficient control mechanism, resulting in elevated serum cholesterol levels, particularly people with *familial hypercholesterolemia* (FH) of genetic origin. Individuals with FH lack the receptors necessary for removing excess cholesterol from the bloodstream and, therefore, exhibit blood cholesterol levels much higher than average.

Nevertheless, the nature of our food can influence the rate of cholesterol synthesis in the liver, as this substance is synthesized mainly from carbohydrates and fats. Clinical studies have shown that the ingestion of sucrose (common table sugar and honey) and fructose (fruit sugar) can increase blood cholesterol levels, as well as the ingestion of hydrogenated vegetable oils that contain harmful artificial *trans* fats. Excess saturated fats can also increase serum cholesterol levels, although each person responds differently to saturated fats.

> Only about 20% to 30% of the serum cholesterol comes from the cholesterol present in food.

Practically, a great part of the foods we ingest can supply the building blocks for cholesterol synthesis, because the liver acts as an efficient biochemical transformation factory.

From a quantitative point of view, the main stream of cholesterol metabolism is its conversion to bile acids in the liver. Part of the bile acids (about 0.8mmoles a day) used in the emulsification of fats for digestion and absorption each day is lost in the feces, and to maintain a constant

> The nature of our food can influence the rate of cholesterol synthesis in the liver.

reservoir (about 15g to 30g) of bile acids, the liver synthesizes those substances from cholesterol.

The ingestion of soluble fibers can reduce the reabsorption of bile acids in the small intestine and their reconversion into cholesterol. To compensate for these losses, more cholesterol needs to be converted into bile acids in the liver. Soluble fibers also promote good intestinal health and physical exercise helps reduce excess cholesterol.

It is believed that excess cholesterol in the bloodstream, especially when oxidized, may damage the cardiovascular system lining (artery walls). Antioxidant substances and protective vitamins such as C and E play an important role in the prevention of atherosclerosis, as they prevent oxidation of bloodstream cholesterol. Research indicates that it is the oxidized cholesterol (damaged by free radicals), not the cholesterol itself, that can harm the artery lining and promote atherosclerosis.

9.3 CHOLESTEROL BIOSYNTHESIS

*C*holesterol is produced in the liver from a substance called *acetyl-coenzyme A* (acetyl-CoA) in a complex series of biochemical reactions and with the participation of several intermediate substances. The liver is the main location of cholesterol synthesis, but the intestine is also relevant. Cholesterol is also synthesized in glands that produce the steroid hormones, such as the adrenal cortex, testicles, and ovaries.

The substratum for cholesterol synthesis (acetyl-CoA) results from the metabolism of organic fuel molecules, mainly carbohydrates and fats, and some amino acids. Acetyl-CoA is a two-carbon molecule, sometimes referred to as the building block of life. In this process, three acetyl-CoA molecules combine to

> The ingestion of soluble fibers can reduce the reabsorption of bile acids in the small intestine and their reconversion into cholesterol.

form an intermediate six-carbon substance called *hydroxy-methyl glutaric acid* (HMG).

The biosynthesis of cholesterol is regulated in a balanced way that depends on the amount captured from food and the concentration of intracellular cholesterol. Less cholesterol is synthesized when the diet contains appropriate amounts of cholesterol. This happens because the biosynthesis in the liver is inhibited by reduced production of the enzyme HMG-CoA (*beta-hydroxy-beta-methylglutaryl-coenzyme A*) reductase. HMG-CoA reductase is a complex regulating enzyme that catalyzes the conversion of HMG-CoA into *mevalonate* (another intermediate step in cholesterol synthesis). Synthesis of this enzyme is inhibited by high levels of intracellular cholesterol and is regulated by hormones and other factors. Evidence indicates that its activity can be varied by a factor as great as 100. Some drugs for cholesterol reduction called *statins* work by inhibiting the production of this enzyme. Statin drugs bring potentially harmful side effects, because they inhibit not just the production of cholesterol but of a whole family of intermediate substances in the mevalonate chemical chain that play important biochemical functions in the body.

> Some drugs for cholesterol reduction works by inhibiting the production of the enzyme HMG-CoA that catalyzes the synthesis of cholesterol in the liver.

The production of cholesterol is also regulated by the hormones *glucagon* and *insulin*, secreted by the pancreas. The enzyme HMG-CoA reductase exists in phosphorylated (inactive) and dephosphorylated (active) forms. Glucagon stimulates *phosphorylation* (inactivation) of the enzyme HMG-CoA reductase, while insulin promotes *dephosphorylation*, activating the enzyme and favoring the synthesis of cholesterol. The insulin and glucagon levels in the blood depend in great part on the amount of carbohydrates and proteins from food, as mentioned in previous chapters. Carbohydrates stimulate the production of insulin (favoring cholesterol

> Cholesterol synthesis is also regulated by the hormones insulin and glucagon, and their blood levels depend on the amount of carbohydrates and proteins from food.

synthesis), whereas proteins favor the secretion of glucagon. Besides reducing cholesterol synthesis, protein helps to burn available body fat and develop lean muscle mass.

9.4 LIPOPROTEINS: THE BLOOD CARRIERS OF CHOLESTEROL

*C*holesterol and the synthesized cholesterol esters, together with other lipids, are transported in the bloodstream through the *plasmatic lipoproteins*. Most of the cholesterol circulating in the blood is not free but is bound to molecules of certain proteins in the serum, forming the lipoprotein particles. Blood, in its bulk part, is essentially an aqueous medium, and the transport of fat molecules (insoluble in water) in the bloodstream is done through the lipoprotein particles, which consist of packages, or molecule aggregates, of cholesterol and various lipid molecules, involved by proteins. The *lipo* (fat soluble) *protein* (water soluble) is, therefore, a substance assembled by the liver (or the intestines) that transports fat-soluble vitamins, cholesterol, and other lipids in the bloodstream. Those particles, or complex molecule aggregates, possess several sizes, compositions, and densities. They are easily mixed with the blood and are transported to the body's tissues and captured by the cells in a process mediated by receptor elements on the cellular membranes.

Plasmatic lipoproteins are surrounded by specific carrier proteins, called *apolipoproteins* or simply *apoproteins* (*apo* designates the protein in its lipid-free form), attached to various combinations of phospholipids, cholesterol, cholesterol esters, and triglycerides. They consist basically of almost globular (spherical) aggregates with the hydrophobic (insoluble in water) lipids in the central core (essentially triglycerides and cholesterol esters), surrounded by a shell composed of cholesterol, phospholipids, and lateral chains of the polar hydrophilic (soluble in water) protein amino acids on the surface. All

> Lipoproteins are almost globular molecule aggregates of cholesterol and various lipid molecules, surrounded by proteins. Different combinations of lipids and proteins produce many kinds of lipoproteins that have different densities and sizes.

lipoproteins have proteins attached to their outer surface, which is how receptors on cells throughout the body recognize them.

Different combinations of lipids and proteins produce many kinds of lipoproteins, which have different sizes and densities varying from relatively very-low to very-high densities. The various lipoproteins can be separated among themselves through ultracentrifugation of blood samples and can be seen with electronic microscopy.

9.5 LIPOPROTEIN STRUCTURE

Lipoproteins are usually classified in terms of the relative amount of fats and proteins they contain. Those that contain relatively more protein and less fat are heavier and denser than those with more fat than protein. The lipoprotein particles are usually classified according to their density ranges:

> High-density lipoproteins (HDL).

> Low-density lipoproteins (LDL).

> Intermediate-density lipoproteins (IDL).

> Very-low density lipoproteins (VLDL).

> Chylomicron.

The term *chylo* here refers to the liquid (with a milky appearance) that contains emulsified fats and is produced during intestinal absorption of emulsified fats from the digestion of foods.

Therefore, the different density ranges refer to their relative content of lipids and proteins. The HDL particles have a larger ratio of proteins (water-soluble elements) to lipids (hydrophobic elements) and are smaller and denser as compared to the LDL particles. Their different content levels of proteins and lipids also act as an address label, allowing the bloodstream to deliver these fat carriers to specific

> The various lipoprotein densities refer to the different proportions of protein and fat that constitute the lipoprotein.

tissues of the body.

Table 9.1 shows the average lipid and protein composition of the main classes of lipoproteins circulating in the blood. Lipoproteins become less dense as their size increases. LDL is about double the size of HDL, whereas VLDL is about six to seven times larger than HDL, in terms of diameter. The chylomicron particles are about 100 times larger than HDL. Figure 9.2 compares, in a simplified way, the relative sizes and compositions of lipoproteins.

TABLE 9.1 – Percent average composition of proteins and lipids of the main lipoprotein classes in the bloodstream and their characteristics.

COMPOSITION	Chylomicron	VLDL	IDL	LDL	HDL
Proteins (S)	1.5-2.5	5-10	15-20	20-25	40-55
Triglycerides (I)	84-89	50-65	22	7-10	3-5
Free cholesterol (S)	1-3	5-10	8	7-10	3-4
Cholesterol esters(I)	3-5	10-15	30	35-40	12
Phospholipids (S)	7-9	15-20	22	15-20	20-35

CHARACTERISTICS	Chylomicron	VLDL	IDL	LDL	HDL
Density (g/cm^3)	< 0.95	< 1.006	1.006-1.019	1.019-1.063	1.063-11.210
Diameter (Angström)	750-12,000	300-800	250-350	180-250	50-120
Mass (kDalton)	400,000	10,000-80,000	5,000-10,000	2,300	175-360

Note: The Dalton is a molecular mass unit equivalent to 1/12 the mass of the isotope 12 of the carbon atom; 1 Angström represents 10^{-10} m.
(S) – Surface component.
(I) – Internal component.

A schematic diagram illustrating the form of the LDL particle, which is the main carrier of cholesterol in the bloodstream, is shown in Figure 9.3. The spherical LDL particle contains about 1,500 molecules of triglycerides and cholesterol esters, covered by an amphiphilic layer of about 800 phospholipid molecules and about 500 cholesterol molecules plus one single apolipoprotein molecule denominated B-100. Table 9.2 shows the physiological functions of the blood lipoproteins and their main origin from the body's tissues.

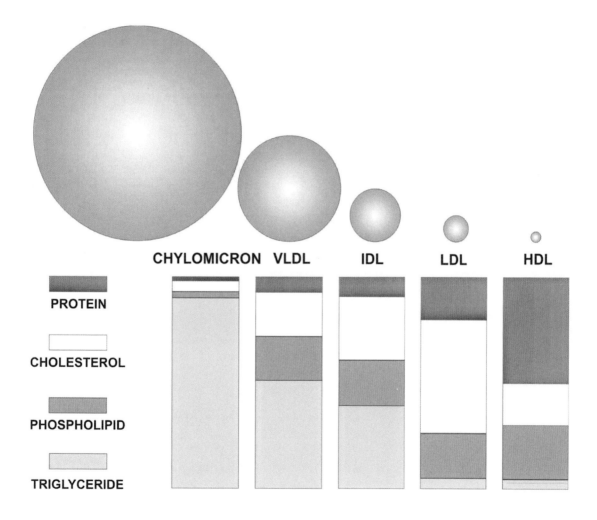

FIGURE 9.2 – Simplified comparison of the relative sizes and compositions of lipoproteins. LDL is about double the size of HDL. VLDL is about six to seven times larger than HDL, whereas the chylomicron particles are approximately 100 times larger than HDL (in terms of diameter).

The chylomicron particle, the largest of all lipoproteins, is formed in the intestinal tract and is filled up mainly with triglycerides (after a meal) alongside a relatively small amount of cholesterol. It travels directly to fat cells in the body without passing through the liver and delivers triglycerides to the cells. In doing so, the chylomicron shrivels into a remnant that is then processed by the liver.

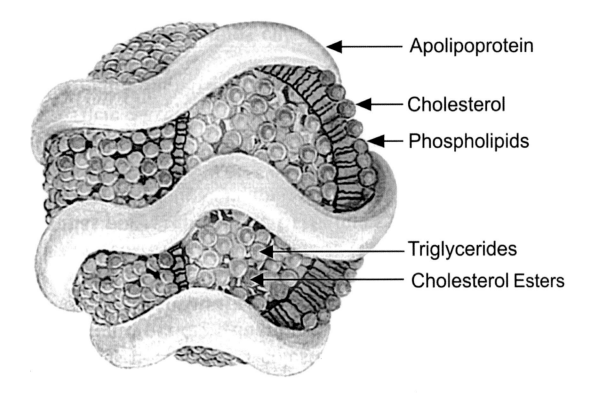

FIGURE 9.3 – Schematic diagram illustrating the LDL particle, which is the main carrier of cholesterol in the bloodstream. Through a 90° cut in the right-hand side, the internal elements (triglycerides and cholesterol esters) and the surface elements (cholesterol and phospholipids) are shown, surrounded by a protein molecule.

The VLDLs are smaller than the chylomicron particles and are manufactured in both the intestines and the liver. They are also composed mainly of triglycerides (see Table 9.1). These two lipoproteins constitute a major part of the fat circulating in the blood. The triglycerides are fundamental for good health, because they constitute a metabolic energy source for the cells. Nevertheless, it is believed that they may be potentially harmful to the arteries when present in excess.

The IDLs are smaller than the VLDLs, and are formed when a VLDL particle delivers triglycerides to the cells and shrinks. When IDL particles shrink to even smaller sizes, they become the LDLs.

> The very-low density lipoproteins (VLDL) are produced in both the intestines and the liver, and are composed mainly of triglycerides.

LDL particles, which also contain relatively more lipids than proteins, deliver cholesterol to the body's tissues and, under certain conditions, they may deliver excessive quantities. When the bloodstream contains many of these particles, they can accumulate at some locations, especially in the cells that cover the blood vessels. Because LDL has more elements of the fatty type, it is more susceptible to oxidation, especially if it contains vegetable oils that can be easily oxidized and does not contain antioxidant substances (such as vitamin E). Once in the cells of the artery walls, LDL can be damaged by highly reacting free radicals, turning into oxidized LDL. Blood white cells attack these deposits of oxidized cholesterol, generating a cascade of reactions that may lead to the accumulation of fatty material (fibrous

> The low-density lipoproteins (LDL) contain more lipids than proteins and may deliver excess cholesterol to the tissues. They are popularly called bad cholesterol.

tissue, cholesterol, debris, and other substances) in the artery walls, eventually leading to the narrowing and hardening of the arteries (atherosclerosis) and reducing blood flow. For these reasons, LDL particles are popularly called *bad cholesterol*.

LDL and VLDL in excess also enhance blood coagulation, which exposes the cardiovascular system to diseases and disorders. Therefore, it is believed that LDL and VLDL, when present in excessive amounts, constitute a risk factor to the cardiovascular system.

HDL particles, which contain relatively more proteins and fewer lipids than LDLs, are smaller and denser than LDL particles. Together with lecithin (phospholipid), they help to remove and eliminate excess cholesterol eventually left by LDL particles. Like a sponge, HDL particles absorb excess cholesterol from the artery walls and other places, and they carry it to other tissues that may need cholesterol or to the liver, where it is reprocessed and converted to bile acids (stored in the gallbladder), which are then eliminated through the bile duct for emulsification and digestion of food fat. They also help the liver to recycle other lipoprotein particles. For these reasons, HDL particles are popularly called *good cholesterol.*

> The high-density lipoproteins (HDL) remove, like a sponge, excess cholesterol eventually left by LDL particles. They are popularly called good cholesterol.

TABLE 9.2 – Main physiological functions of the blood lipoproteins and their main origin from the body's tissues.

CLASS	ORIGIN	PHYSIOLOGICAL FUNCTION
Chylomicron	Intestine	Absorption of fats from the diet.
Fragments of Chylomicron	Plasma	Delivers fats from the diet to the liver.
VLDL	Liver	Transports triglycerides from the liver to other tissues.
IDL	Plasma	Initial products formed from VLDL catabolism.
LDL	Plasma	Transports cholesterol esters.
HDL	Liver and Intestine	Removes excess cholesterol from tissues and lipoproteins, and remodels lipoproteins.

It is important to emphasize that cholesterol is essential for good health and that there is no such thing as a "bad" molecular type, or a "good" molecular type of cholesterol. The terminology may be confusing and is, of course, inadequate. The difference between what is popularly called good and bad cholesterol lies in the density and composition (relative amounts of cholesterol, lipids, and proteins) of the lipoproteins that transport the cholesterol molecules and other lipids in the bloodstream to the tissues.

An appropriate balance between LDL and HDL lipoproteins is therefore fundamental to maintain adequate cholesterol levels in the bloodstream and for good health, as well as the presence of adequate levels of fat-soluble antioxidants such as vitamin E. Vitamin E constitutes the primary protector against the oxidative damages to LDL particles. Ideally, about one-third of the total of lipoproteins in the bloodstream should be in the form HDL.

According to research, people who accumulate body fat mainly in the abdominal area (popularly called *apple shape*) have levels of HDL lower than those with fat accumulation predominantly in the hips (*pear shape*). This is because fat in the hips tends to be subcutaneous, whereas fat around the waist is intra-abdominal, so it drains directly to the liver and interferes with the liver production of HDL. Premenopausal women usually have higher levels of HDL than men in the same age range. The artificial trans fats (usually present in partially hydrogenated vegetable oils or vegetable fats), as well as saturated fats when consumed in excess, have been associated with high LDL blood levels.

> Ideally, about one-third of the total of lipoproteins in the bloodstream should be in the form HDL.

9.6 SUB-FRACIONS OF LDL PARTICLES

Cholesterol is an essential metabolic nutrient and one of the body's most vital molecules. It produces vitamin D, adrenal and sexual hormones, bile salts for digestion, and creates neurotransmission impulses in the brain. In fact, the higher your cholesterol, the longer you will live. It is a life-sustaining molecule.

Cholesterol has no direct correlation with heart disease risk and may become only dangerous when oxidation and inflammation occur due to poor diet (when you eat lots of sugar and glycemic carbohydrates) and poor exercise habits. The true heart disease risk factors (oxidation and inflammation) are driven strongly by polyunsaturated and trans fats, simple sugars and glycemic carbohydrates, excess insulin production and emotional stress. They are inflammatory to the endothelium cells. Limiting sugars and glycemic carbohydrates and eating more high quality fats and whole foods (including saturated animal fat and eggs, in moderation) can promote health, weight management, and reduced risk of heart disease. Actually, saturated fat is our preferred fuel and has no direct correlation with heart disease risk. Saturated animal fat is a major dietary calorie source (from animal foods) and drove human evolution/advancement of brain function for two million years. In moderation, it promotes efficient fat metabolism, weight control and stable energy levels.

The total blood cholesterol number may be mostly meaningless without further context. Nevertheless, compiling all the possible figures can provide clues to your heart health. The triglyceride to HDL ratio is a good indicator and a ratio of 3:1 or less is recommended, while less than 2 is considered outstanding for heart health. A favourable ratio indicates that you have plenty of HDL particles to scavenge the bloodstream for potentially damaging agents. Triglycerides exceeding 150mg/dl indicates more oxidized LDL and thus poor health and elevated heart disease risk. Strive to get triglycerides below 100mg/dl and HDL above 50mg/dl. This may be the best of the old cholesterol science (last century).

The new science considers cholesterol fractionization, since not all LDL particles are inflammatory to the endothelium cells and atherogenic, but only the smaller and denser ones, as well as the small Lp(a) particles that make the blood clot and cause inflammation inside the blood vessels. Lp(a) is another key inflammation marker associated with small, dense LDL particles. The larger and fluffy LDL particles seem not to be a problem. Therefore, total blood LDL values offer better context when particle sizes and sub-fractions are identified, since only small, dense LDL particles should be of any concern. A preponderance of small and dense LDL particles in the profile can indicate poor LDL clearance from blood and greater chance of oxidation, inflammation, and potential damage to the cardiovascular system. Thus, laboratory tests for blood cholesterol (i.e. lipoproteins), to be meaningful, should dissect and fractionate the total LDL in terms of particle sizes and densities.

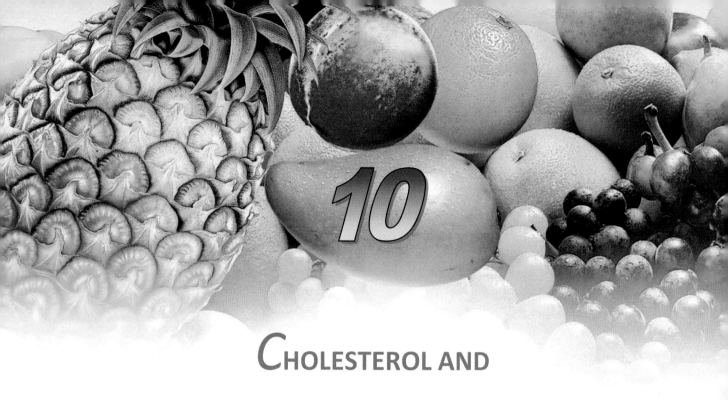

CHOLESTEROL AND

CARDIOVASCULAR HEALTH

10.1 LOW-FAT DIETS

*C*ontrary to popular belief, a low-fat diet actually increases the risk of cardiovascular disease. Research has shown that low-fat diets have a negative effect on the blood lipoprotein profile and on the cardiovascular system for complex reasons that may depend partly on genetic differences. In fat-restricted diets, the body begins to produce a greater number of smaller and denser LDL particles, considered potentially much more inflammatory and harmful when compared to the larger and less-dense ones, increasing the risk of cardiovascular disease. A low-fat diet also reduces the blood level of HDLs, which help to remove excess cholesterol, further worsening the problem.

Many low-fat diets are compensated by a greater ingestion of carbohydrates, which increases the blood levels of insulin, triglycerides, cholesterol, and VLDL. These diets enhance the risk of developing cardiovascular disease and cause abrupt variations in the blood levels of glucose and insulin, which may lead to obesity and diabetes.

> Low-fat diets have a negative effect on the blood lipoprotein profile and on the cardiovascular system.

Another effect of a low-fat diet is increased levels of a blood lipoprotein called lipoprotein-(a), or Lp(a), which is considered inflammatory and harmful to the cardiovascular system. Lp(a) is actually another form of LDL, the difference being that it has two types of proteins attached to the outside. Research indicates that the artificial trans fats present in partially hydrogenated vegetable oils (margarine, for instance) increase blood levels of Lp(a), whereas saturated fats reduce them.

Fat-soluble vitamins (A, D, E, and K), as well as many fat-soluble antioxidant substances (beta-carotene and lycopene, for instance) are appropriately absorbed in the body only when ingested with fatty foods.

Evidence gathered in the second half of the last century, however, indicates that the increase in cardiovascular disease occurrence is clearly correlated with the increase (in the last several decades) in consumption of sugars, refined carbohydrates, refined delicate vegetable oils, oxidized oils (as in fried foods), hydrogenated vegetable oils (containing trans fats), and industrialized foods that contain these ingredients.

> A low-fat diet actually increases the risk of cardiovascular disease and, when compensated with a larger ingestion of carbohydrates, may lead to obesity and diabetes.

As discussed in the chapter on fatty acids and health, saturated fats are not intrinsically harmful and constitute a fundamental part of body metabolism. Fat synthesized in the liver occurs in the saturated form and is incorporated in the glycerol chemical structure in the form of triglycerides. Saturated fats have been linked to cardiovascular disease only when they are consumed in excess and as part of an unbalanced diet, deficient in nutrients and antioxidants, that includes excess calories, sugar, refined carbohydrates, and that is altered by free radicals generated by body metabolism. The presence of toxins in food and in the environment also plays a part. Excess glycemic carbohydrates in the diet negatively affect the normal metabolism of saturated fats.

10.2 ATHEROSCLEROSIS AND HEART DISEASE

*M*any factors can contribute to the development of cardiovascular disease, such as high blood pressure, diabetes, excess blood cholesterol (oxidized), and genetic predisposition. Factors related to lifestyle (cigarette smoking, obesity, sedentary behavior, inadequate eating habits, physical and emotional stress, toxic substances in foods and the environment) may also increase the risk. However, none of those risks, or a combination of them, guarantees that someone will develop cardiovascular disease. According to research, a large number of people with high blood cholesterol levels, for instance, do not die from heart disease. Nevertheless, it is necessary for preventive purposes to take all these factors into account.

What is often called heart disease is not truly a disease of the heart but of the arteries that supply blood and oxygen to the heart. The arteries are essential to feed each organ's cells with blood rich in oxygen and nutrients. The *coronary arteries* exercise a crucial role, because they feed the heart muscle itself (see Figure 10.1). Without a constant flow of blood through the coronary arteries, the heart muscle weakens and, without oxygen, some of its cells may die.

Coronary heart disease (CHD) initially consists of a chronic phase: during the development of atherosclerosis, *plaque* (a grey-white/fatty gunk) builds up on the artery walls over many years. It is essentially the result of an inflammatory immune response to arterial injury, not simply the product of blood cholesterol elevation. The body's response to arterial damage involves inflammation, so atherosclerosis is an *inflammatory disorder*. Cholesterol supplies all-important structural integrity to the cell membranes, and as part of the body's attempt to repair a damaged section of artery, the body channels cholesterol into areas of the artery with a high proportion of damaged cells. Cholesterol

> The coronary arteries play a crucial role in heart disease, because they feed the heart muscle itself.

will not accumulate within artery walls that are not damaged.

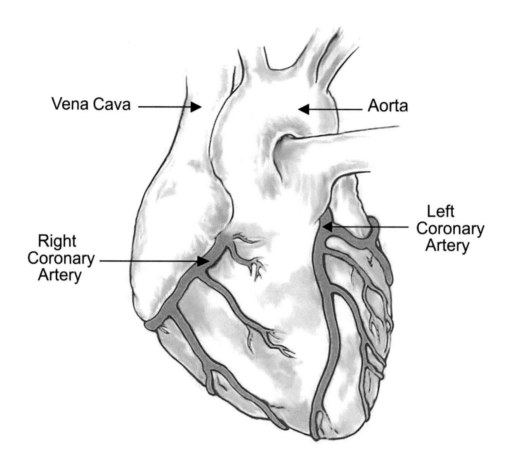

FIGURE 10.1 – Illustrating the coronary arteries that feed the heart muscle. The *aorta* conducts oxygen-rich blood to the body, and the *vena cava* returns blood to the heart.

Excess LDL in the blood constitutes only a part of the cardiovascular problem, because it becomes a threat only when it is oxidized, or damaged by free radicals, and begins to form deposits on the artery walls. Those lipid deposits (particularly cholesterol esters) happen initially inside the cells of the arterial smooth musculature and of *macrophages*. At this stage, the deposits of oxidized lipids are reversible and may not result in permanent damage to the artery wall. Those recent lesions are called *fatty patches*. White cells in the blood attack these plaques, generating fragments or debris, at the same time that the arterial wall cells try to cure themselves by developing new cells in the walls.

The accumulation of oxidized fatty plaques, debris, and fibrous tissue of additional cells causes narrowing and hardening of the arteries and restrict blood flow (see Figure 10.2). The continued development of plaque causes thickening of the artery wall, which leads to a loss of elasticity. Eventually, the plaques can reach the stage in which they actually calcify, turning the arteries into stiff, almost bone-like tubes. At advanced stages, additional fatty and fibrous deposits produce an *atheroma*, which is a bulged plaque build-up within the artery wall formed of a mixture of collagen, calcium, arterial muscle cells, white blood cells, blood platelets, fatty acids, and cholesterol and often covered by a fibrous cap.

> Atherosclerosis is essentially a process in which plaque forms inside the arteries over many years, and it is not simply the product of blood cholesterol elevation, but an inflammatory immune response to arterial injury.

The development of atherosclerosis may not produce any symptoms until a heart attack or cerebral hemorrhage (a stroke) occurs. Heart strokes are caused by an insufficient amount of blood feeding the heart muscle or by a serious irregularity in the heart beat frequency (*spasms*). The heart signals insufficient blood supply through severe chest pain (*angina*).

Coronary events (the acute phase of coronary heart disease) may occur when a narrowed section of artery undergoes spasm and blocks blood flow to the heart, or when an unstable plaque or fibrous scar tissue covering an atheroma ruptures. In the latter instance, the atheroma contents spill into the bloodstream, causing the blood to rapidly clot. These blood clots (*thrombi*) may completely block the artery at the rupture site, or they may break away and travel through the bloodstream, eventually blocking another area narrowed by plaque.

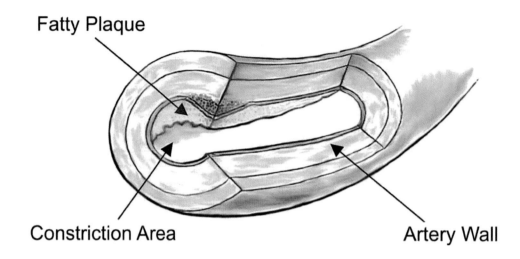

FIGURE 10.2 – Plaque formation due to deposits of oxidized fatty material and debris in the lining of the artery internal walls, which narrow the artery cross-section and stiffen the artery walls.

If a coronary artery with an already restricted cross-section is completely blocked by a blood clot (*thrombus*), the heart muscle is denied the oxygen and nutrient-rich blood that it needs to keep pumping, resulting in a *coronary thrombosis*. Part of the heart muscle tissue may die due to lack of blood and oxygen. The result is a heart attack, also called a *myocardial infarction*. If the area of dead heart muscle is small, the damage may not be fatal. The area heals, forming a hard fibrous tissue, and the recovery may be complete. The heart may eventually grow new arteries to bypass the blockage (collateral circulation), or the blocked artery may reopen.

Heart strokes are caused by an insufficient amount of blood feeding the heart muscle or by a serious irregularity in the heart beat frequency (spasms).

If thrombosis occurs in the brain arteries, part of the brain cells may die, leading to an *ischemic stroke*. *Hemorrhagic stroke* is a different process, in which blood vessels in the brain rupture, flooding surrounding tissues with blood and eventually causing the death of some brain cells.

Blood is normally a slippery fluid. In the case of a cut or wound, blood platelets adhere to each other and start the coagulation process. The tendency of coagulation of the blood can be specified by a parameter called the *index of adhesion* of the platelets. A healthy person usually possesses an index around 20 (that is, the blood is not sticky). This index is measured by passing blood through a small glass tube in an instrument, where the number 20 means that 20% of the blood platelets adhere to the tube walls. Measurements made involving people who suffered a heart attack show an index of about 90 (that is, a blood with a high tendency to coagulate).

The cells in the artery walls usually produce *prostacyclin* (or prostaglandin PGI_2), a substance that prevents blood platelets from adhering to each other and to the artery walls. However, arteries damaged by fatty deposits, plaques, and high blood pressure do not normally produce appropriate amounts of this prostaglandin. As explained in the chapter on fatty acids and health, the prostaglandins PGE_1 and PGE_3, produced from some fatty acids (GLA, and EPA and DHA, respectively) can reduce the tendency of blood platelet aggregation.

Therefore, the ingestion of GLA from primrose and borage oils, as well as the ingestion of EPA and DHA, found primarily in fish oils, helps in the maintenance of slippery and less-viscous blood and in preventing clot formation. Besides primrose, borage, and fish oils, vitamin E is also of great importance in protecting against cardiovascular disease, because it protects the lipids in the LDL particle from oxidation, combats free radicals, increases HDL blood levels, and helps in the formation of prostacyclin (PGI_2), which reduces blood platelet aggregation. Aspirin also has an efficient blood-thinning effect and can be almost as effective as drugs designed to break down blood clots, besides having an important anti-inflammatory effect on the cardiovascular system.

> The ingestion of the fatty acids GLA (from primrose and borage oils) and EPA and DHA (from fish oils) helps in the maintenance of slippery and less-viscous blood.

Another type of heart attack is caused by arterial spasms, mainly in arteries already partially damaged by fatty deposits. The artery walls can contract vigorously as a result of a serious wound, tension, or emotional shock. The mechanism involved in those spasms is well known, and the tension or emotional shock induces the nerves to release substances that cause the artery to constrict. The blood flow reduction also decreases the oxygen available to the arterial muscle. If the decrease is small, the artery relaxes, but if the supply of oxygen is drastically diminished, the heart muscle may suffer spasms. Cigarette smokers already have a reduced availability of oxygen, so the combination of tension and cigarettes may be fatal in many occasions. During arterial spasms, PGI_2 is not released, while PGE_2 (which increases the coagulation tendency) can be. Consequently, the blood platelets tend to stick to each other and to the artery walls, forming clots that block the flow of blood.

> The combination of stress and cigarette smoking may be fatal in many occasions.

10.3 CHOLESTEROL OXIDATION

Cholesterol is found in every cell. Without it, the body cannot produce hormones, vitamin D, and cell membranes. It is constantly present in the bloodstream and becomes potentially harmful only when oxidized or damaged. The evidence accumulated in the last few decades indicates that the stiffening and narrowing of arteries are consequences of damages induced by oxidized cholesterol, not by cholesterol itself.

The level of oxidation that the lipids, present in the lipoproteins, may suffer depends on the following factors:

➢ Susceptibility of oxidation of the fatty acids present in the lipoprotein particle.

➢ The amount and balance of antioxidant substances (such as vitamin E) present in the lipoprotein particle.

➢ The amount of free radicals in the body.

The increased occurrence of heart disease during the last century is basically due to a fundamentally unbalanced diet: essential vitanutrients are removed in processed foods, and excessive consumption of sugars, refined carbohydrates, refined and oxidized vegetable oils, and hydrogenated vegetable oils (containing trans fats) all negatively affect body metabolism and its ability to correctly process cholesterol.

Part of the problem starts with the generation of free radicals that oxidize cholesterol, damaging it and giving rise to plaque formation in the arteries and inflammation. Free radicals are unstable compounds generated as by-products of body metabolism or from toxic substances and stress. They are highly reactive molecular fragments in search of chemical stability. When the body is well-nourished, free radicals are neutralized by certain vitanutrients and enzymes known as antioxidants.

> Cholesterol is constantly present in the bloodstream and becomes potentially harmful only when oxidized or damaged.

Vitamin E, which is fat-soluble, is as an excellent antioxidant that protects against cardiovascular disease and other illnesses. Other important antioxidants are vitamin C, vitamin B_5 (pantothenic acid), beta-carotene, and lycopene. A low level of vitamin E in the blood may be considered a risk factor as important as high serum cholesterol.

It is important to avoid oxidized oils, which are free-radical generators. The stability of the LDL particle against oxidation depends on the susceptibility to oxidation of the lipids present in the food. Refined PUFAs commonly used for cooking, such as soy, corn, and sunflower oils, are very delicate and easily oxidized, particularly when heated to high temperatures, and they constitute a risk. The refinement process removes the natural antioxidants, leaving them still more fragile. When incorporated into LDL particles, these oils leave the cholesterol subject to oxidation, thus increasing the risk of cardiovascular disease. Oils

> Free radicals are unstable compounds generated as by-products of body metabolism, or from toxic substances and stress.

rich in MUFAs such as extra virgin olive and canola oils, as well as saturated fats, are much more stable and less subject to oxidation and will promote the stability of the cholesterol when incorporated into the LDL particle. Macadamias and peanuts are also rich in MUFAs.

Fried foods of any type constitute a great risk, because oils heated to high temperatures for a long time become highly oxidized, generating chemical substances called *lipid peroxides*. Those peroxides are highly reactive and may cause cardiovascular disease and cancer. Stir-frying foods does not seem to pose the same risks.

The ingestion of foods that contain oxidized cholesterol, such as matured fatty meats, is not advisable. These meats possess a high content of toxins (as *malonaldeid*) and carcinogenic substances. Some aged fatty cheeses may also contain oxidized cholesterol. Though they are rich in cholesterol, eggs are good foods, and countless studies have indicated that eggs do not increase the risk of cardiovascular disease. However, powdered eggs (that include the yolk) found in mixtures for cakes and other industrialized products should be avoided, because they may contain oxidized cholesterol. Powdered integral milks may also contain oxidized cholesterol. Fresh meats, poultry, fish, non-aged cheeses, yogurts, and eggs do not contain oxidized cholesterol and may be consumed. They are excellent sources of complete proteins and other nutrients.

> Fried foods constitute a great risk for cardiovascular disease, because oils heated to high temperatures for a long time become highly oxidized, generating potentially harmful lipid peroxides.

It is also important to avoid oxidizing substances present in the environment and those generated from lifestyle and stress. Cigarette smoking (or inhaling second-hand smoke) is an unhealthy source of oxidizing chemical substances, as well as many chemical substances added to processed foods such as salami and sausages, exposure to radiation and ultraviolet light, and excessive practice of stressful aerobic exercises that enhance oxidative metabolism.

Steps to prevent cardiovascular disease should include the elimination of all processed and refined foods and reducing sources of free radicals from the diet, lifestyle, and environment. We must also supply the body with a powerful arsenal of free-radical fighting antioxidants and nutrients that deliver as many protective vitamins, minerals, trace elements, amino acids, and phytochemicals per ingested calorie as possible.

10.4 NUTRIENTS AND CARDIOVASCULAR HEALTH

*T*he interactions between food nutrients and the cardiovascular system are extensive and complex, and numerous *non-drug* measures can reduce the risk of coronary heart disease. The benefits provided by healthy food, vitamins, antioxidants, physical exercise, and stress avoidance must be emphasized.

Fresh vegetables and fruits, in general, provide valuable nutrients such as folic acid, vitamin C, carotenoids such as alpha-carotene, beta-carotene, lycopene, cryptoxanthin, and lutein, and countless phytochemical substances (such as polyphenols and bioflavonoids) that possess remarkable antioxidant and disease-fighting properties. Nuts (such as almonds, macadamias, cashews, pecans, walnuts, pistachios, and Brazil nuts) and seeds (sesame, sunflower, pumpkin, and flax) are excellent sources of important minerals such as magnesium and selenium, vitamin E, healthy fats, and some amino acids.

> To avoid coronary heart disease we must supply the body with a powerful arsenal of free-radical fighting antioxidant nutrients that deliver as many protective vitamins, minerals, trace elements, amino acids, and phytochemicals per ingested calorie as possible.

Selenium and vitamins A, C, and E act as antioxidants that prevent free-radical damage to the artery walls and heart. Vitamin C, copper, and the amino acids proline and lysine are necessary for healthy formation of collagen, which literally holds the arteries together. Magnesium, co-enzyme Q_{10}, L-carnitine, and taurine play important roles in energy production and muscular contraction, and they are essential for healthy cardiac function.

Arginine is necessary for adequate *nitric oxide* (NO) release in the arteries, which is essential for proper artery expansion and contraction and cardiovascular function. The richest source of the amino acid arginine is peanuts.

> There are many non-drug measures that can reduce the risk of cardiovascular disease.

Peanuts should not be eaten raw but slightly toasted (avoid salted peanuts toasted in vegetable fat). The hull of some nuts and seeds may contain small amounts of *phytates*, an antinutrient substance that is also present in similar amounts in grains and legumes, but the nutritional qualities of nuts and seeds are far superior to that of cereal grains.

Omega-3 fatty acids from fish, or fish oil supplements, and flaxseed help to prevent inflammation, the formation of blood clots, and potentially fatal heartbeat irregularities.

> Vitamins A, C, and E, and selenium act as antioxidants that prevent free-radical damage to the arteries and heart.

It is important to maintain blood glucose levels within the normal range. The simple but most effective strategy for lowering elevated blood glucose and triglyceride levels is to drastically reduce carbohydrate intake. Lowering your blood sugar also lowers free-radical activity. A true low-carbohydrate diet is one that supplies less than 100 grams of carbohydrate per day, preferably ones with a low glycemic index (GI), and that also supply important nutrients. If you intend to reduce your intake of carbohydrates, it is advisable to do so gradually instead of shocking the body with a sharp reduction. Excess carbohydrate consumption, especially of the refined variety, raises blood sugar and insulin levels. It increases the risk of diabetes, accelerates glycation (oxidation of blood proteins), free-radical activity, blood clots, and the proliferation of arterial smooth muscle cells, where plaques tend to develop.

> A simple and effective dietary strategy for lowering elevated blood levels of glucose and triglycerides is to reduce carbohydrate intake.

Avoid low-fat, high-carbohydrate diets and refined polyunsaturated vegetable oils rich in omega-6 fatty acids. These refined oils are highly susceptible to free-radical damage. MUFAs and saturated fatty acids (because of their lack of vulnerable double bonds) are the least susceptible to free-radical damage. Research has consistently shown that low-fat meals drastically reduce the absorption of vitally important fat-soluble vitamins (such as A, D, and E) and carotenoids.

The highest concentrations of fat-soluble vitamins and carotenoids are found in the fatty portions of meat, fish, dairy products, and eggs. Egg yolks and liver beef are especially concentrated dietary sources of lecithin and choline, which are required for healthy liver function, maintenance of brain cell membranes and nerve sheaths (myelin), and the formation of the key neurotransmitter *acetyl-choline*.

Low-fat diets also lower the levels of testosterone, essential for well-being in both men and women, whereas saturated and monounsaturated fats positively influence hormonal function. Free testosterone elevates the sex drive, improves muscle growth, bone density, and immune function and may even protect against cardiovascular disease.

> Avoid low-fat, high-carbohydrate diets and refined polyunsaturated vegetable oils rich in omega-6 fatty acids.

Cardiovascular and coronary diseases occur mainly in groups of people that consume refined foods that are deprived of natural antioxidants. Those foods include sugar (in many forms), white flour (and products that include it), margarine, hydrogenated vegetable oils or vegetable fat, refined vegetable oils that are easily oxidized, industrialized foods that contain these substances, and similar products. A significant portion of the calorie content in many industrialized foods comes from cereal flour (usually refined wheat flour), sugar (in various forms such as syrups, sucrose, fructose, maltodextrin, and dextrose), refined vegetable oils, and hydrogenated vegetable oils or vegetable fat (containing trans fats). These low-nutrient foods (empty calories) should be avoided.

Besides avoiding these substances, maintaining an ideal weight is recommended. We should ingest optimum levels of antioxidant

> Cardiovascular and coronary diseases occur mainly in groups of people that consume refined foods that are deprived of natural antioxidants.

vitanutrients such as vitamins E and C, beta-carotene, and selenium. When taking vitamin E supplements, give preference to a mixed *tocopherol* and *tocotrienol* formula or emphasize foods rich in *gamma-tocopherol*. The best sources of gamma-tocopherol are sesame seeds, pecans, walnuts, pistachios, and pumpkin seeds; cashew nuts and Brazil nuts also contain relatively high amounts. Brazil nuts are particularly rich in selenium.

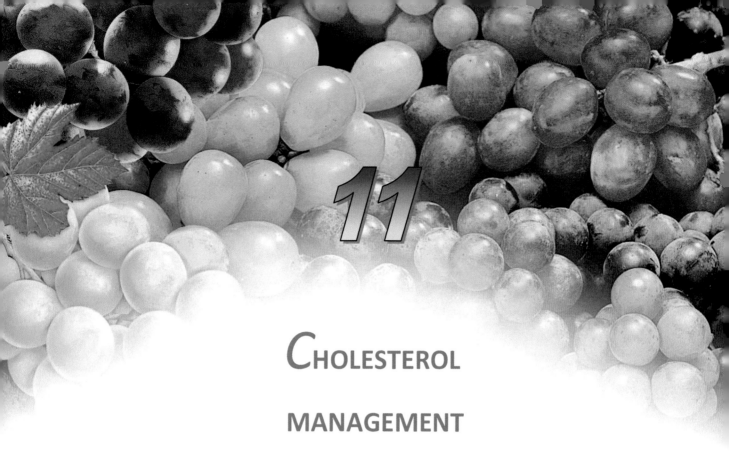

Cholesterol

Management

11.1 NORMALIZING YOUR CHOLESTEROL

When unhealthy eating habits, lack of exercise (sedentary behavior), or genetic tendencies result in LDL excess and HDL deficiency, it becomes necessary to improve the proportion between these blood lipoproteins (that is, to reduce LDL and increase HDL levels). An adequately balanced diet that contains the necessary nutrients, together with physical exercise, leads in this direction. The ratio of HDL to total cholesterol is more relevant than the total amount of cholesterol in the blood. The ideal ratio of HDL to total cholesterol is considered to be approximately 1:3.

Blood cholesterol levels ranging between 160mg/l and 230mg/l are considered normal and necessary for good health. However, high levels of free radicals and oxidizing substances in the body increase the possibility that the cholesterol will become oxidized and contribute to atherosclerosis. Cholesterol in the bloodstream does not constitute a risk as long as it is protected by antioxidant substances such as vitamin E and exists in adequate amounts, with a good proportion of HDL to total cholesterol.

It is fundamental to eliminate from the diet all refined carbohydrates and to restrict, to some extent, the ingestion of carbohydrates in general (even whole ones), in order to lower the blood levels of cholesterol, triglycerides, and insulin. High levels of triglycerides, VLDL, and insulin are a direct consequence of excess ingestion of high-GI carbohydrates. Insulin activates the enzyme HMG-CoA reductase (enzyme necessary for one of the stages of cholesterol biosynthesis), whereas the hormone glucagon disables it, reducing the synthesis of cholesterol. Choose unrefined whole foods as close as possible to their natural state, including adequate amounts of complete proteins, which stimulate the production of glucagon by the pancreas. Avoid trans fats and oils heated to high temperatures for long periods (fried foods), but include appropriate amounts of essential fatty acids and oils that promote a good balance in prostaglandin metabolism (primrose, borage, flaxseed, and fish oils).

> High levels of free radicals and oxidizing substances in the body increase the possibility that cholesterol will become oxidized and contribute to atherosclerosis.

Some vitanutrients may help to reduce blood cholesterol levels. Vitamin B_3 (or niacin) is sometimes effective in reducing cholesterol levels, as well as lecithin combined with vitamin C. Some studies have shown that *pantethine*, a substance derived from pantothenic acid (vitamin B_5), is also effective at lowering excess cholesterol, triglycerides, and other blood lipids. Some complex B vitamins (mainly folic acid, B_6 and B_{12}) help to reduce blood levels of a substance called *homocistein*, an amino acid present in the blood considered to be a risk factor for cardiovascular disease. Magnesium and chromium, as well as the amino acid *L-carnitine*, not only help to reduce total cholesterol but also increase HDL levels. L-carnitine also reduces the blood level of triglycerides. Clinical experiments have shown that chromium can reduce atherosclerotic plaques, and beta-carotene can increase HDL levels.

Garlic, onion, and yogurt (with good-quality *acidophilus*) can reduce cholesterol levels. Virtually all nuts in natural form can reduce cholesterol, as well as the fatty acids in flaxseed, canola oil, and extra-virgin olive oil, GLA in primrose and borage oils, and EPA and DHA in fish oils.

Another way to reduce cholesterol is consuming *phytosterols*, which are sterols found in plants. They are poorly absorbed by humans and are of current interest because they reduce intestinal absorption of cholesterol. They have recently been introduced in some vegetable oil spreads as a cholesterol-lowering ingredient.

The ingestion of soluble fibers, present in many natural foods such as oat bran, soy, flaxseed, apple, carrot, and citric fruits, also helps to reduce blood cholesterol levels, as they prevent the reabsorption of bile acids from the small intestine and their reconversion into cholesterol. Soluble fibers also prevent intestine affections and help to combat Type 2 diabetes. *Pectin*, a soluble fiber present in many fruits and vegetables (carrot and apple, for instance), and the soluble fibers present in vegetables, cereals, nuts, and seeds, all help to reduce serum cholesterol. The soluble fibers contained in grapefruit help reduce blood cholesterol.

> Ingestion of soluble fibers can reduce the reabsorption of bile acids from the small intestine and their reconversion into cholesterol.

11.2 CHOLESTEROL-LOWERING MEDICATION

*T*hough a common practice of modern medicine, the use of medication to reduce high blood cholesterol levels is still controversial, and many researchers affirm that medications should be recommended only in cases of high risk of heart disease and stroke or in familial hypercholesterolemia. Improved eating habits and lifestyle are much more important and may be fundamental to normalize the blood levels of cholesterol. Some of these medications, called *statins*, can produce a variety of negative and insidious side effects, and the health risk from their use must be carefully evaluated on a regular basis.

A plant that grows in China, *red yeast rice*, eventually kills the animals that are foolish enough to eat it. After extensive research, it was discovered that this plant produces a poison called *lovastatin* that inhibits the production of the enzyme HMG-CoA reductase necessary for the biosynthesis of cholesterol; the animals dyed due to problems resulting from lack of cholesterol and side effects. Considering the *cholesterol hypothesis*, which states that excess cholesterol may cause cardiovascular and coronary disease, the pharmaceutical industry decided to use small (non-deadly) doses of this substance to reduce the biosynthesis of cholesterol in human beings.

> Medication to reduce high blood cholesterol levels are currently indicated in cases of high risk of heart disease and stroke or in familial hypercholesterolemia.

Since then, many other types of statins (*simvastatin, pravastatin, fluvastatin, atorvastatin, cerivastatin, and rosuvastatin*) have been patented and produced by the pharmaceutical industry, with impressive financial profits, with the allegation that they reduce cardiovascular and heart disease risk by inhibiting cholesterol biosynthesis. To maintain profits, the pharmaceutical industry initiated a series of controlled experiments in groups of people to show that these drugs really work. One famous American cardiologist, *Robert C. Atkins, M. D.*, stated in one of his many books that he considers statins one of the greatest fiascos of modern medicine, because the drug does not address the real causes that lead to elevated blood cholesterol levels or cardiovascular disease. Other studies questioning the cholesterol hypothesis and the use of statins have been presented and discussed in articles and books by learned cardiologists such as *Anthony Colpo* and *Malcolm Kendrick* (see Bibliography). In fact, *Dr. Kendrick* affirms in his book (*The Great Cholesterol Con*) that the misguided war against cholesterol, using statins, represents something very close to a crime against

> Improved eating habits and lifestyle may be fundamental to normalize blood cholesterol levels.

humanity. There seems to be endless contradictions to the cholesterol hypothesis and there are many hundreds of researchers and doctors that consider it a mistake.

Statins act by inhibiting the production of HMG-CoA reductase. This enzyme is necessary for producing a host of substances (in the same chain of chemical reactions that lead to cholesterol production) that play important biochemical functions in the body, including production of coenzyme Q_{10} (CoQ_{10}), which is essential for supplying energy to the cells and heart muscle. The heart pumps blood through the body at a rate of about 100,000 times per day (approximately seventy times per minute), so it is extremely dependent on CoQ_{10}. Statins may also damage the liver and its metabolism.

> Our heart is extremely dependent on coenzyme Q_{10} in order to pump blood through the body at a rate of about 100,000 times per day.

Countless studies have shown that, except perhaps in individuals with pre-existing coronary heart disease, these drugs seem to reduce lifespan and not the opposite, for various reasons. The drugs do not attack the main causes of cardiovascular disease, which are the nutritional deficiencies, lack of physical exercise, and cellular damage induced by oxidizing substances and free radicals. At the same time, they accelerate present diseases and reduce the energy levels of the heart muscle through inhibition of CoQ_{10} synthesis. Sometimes, the blood cholesterol level rises as an antioxidant defense, and artificially reducing it removes the body's established protection. Instead of using these drugs, options for preventing cardiovascular disease include rational modification of diet and lifestyle, eating vitanutrient supplements, moderate physical exercise, and stress control.

Some studies of lipid-lowering drugs indicate that any association between serum cholesterol and coronary heart disease is secondary at best, and that these drugs may influence heart disease through mechanisms

> There is evidence that statins may exert a variety of small but favorable effects on the cardiovascular system and coronary health, not related to cholesterol reduction.

other than merely lowering cholesterol. There is evidence that statins seem to exert a multitude of small but favorable effects on the cardiovascular system and coronary health that seem to be unrelated to cholesterol reduction, but possibly to anti-inflammatory effects.

Statins seem to improve *endothelial* function and may be beneficial in treating cardiovascular disease. Some of the cardiovascular benefits of the use of statins include anti-inflammatory effects (reduction in C-reactive protein, CRP, a marker of inflammatory activity), anticlotting effects (reduction in blood platelet production of thromboxane, an eicosanoid that stimulates blood clotting), improved arterial function (better endothelial function and blood flow), antioxidant effects (reduced oxidized LDL), reversal or decrease of atherosclerotic plaque formation, inhibition of the migration and proliferation of smooth muscle cells that are seen during atherosclerotic plaque formation, prevention of atherosclerotic plaque rupture, prevention of cardiac hypertrophy, and increased nitric oxide activity (which helps maintain healthy arteries).

> Statins may improve endothelial function and may be beneficial in treating cardiovascular disease.

In some clinical trials, statins have demonstrated the ability (although small) to reduce cardiovascular and overall mortality in individuals with pre-existing coronary heart disease, and they may impart similar benefits to persons with hypertension and diabetes.

11.3 STATIN SIDE EFFECTS

The use of statins, nevertheless, is of considerable risk due to the insidious side effects. People around the world have exposed themselves to the many well-documented side effects of these widely prescribed cholesterol-lowering drugs. Statin users have reported an alarming array of frequent side effects, which are no doubt a major reason why most people taking statins discontinue their use. The most

> Statin drugs can produce a variety of negative and insidious side effects, some of which can be quite harmful.

common side effects are extreme fatigue, muscle weakness and pain, nausea, gastrointestinal problems, liver dysfunctions, lethargy, depression, irritability, dizziness, and cognitive disturbances ranging from confusion to transient amnesia. The dangers from the use of statins are real and may lead to death.

Statins cause muscle pains and muscle weakness in up to 20% of people taking them. Some statins may cause *rhabdomyolysis* or severe muscle damage (disintegration), which releases massive amounts of muscle protein (from death skeletal muscle cells) into the bloodstream. Rhabdomyolysis means the decomposition or break down (suffix *lysis*) of the skeletal muscle (*rhabdomyo*) caused by damages to the muscle tissue. When liver enzyme levels rise, patients must be advised to stop taking the drug or reduce the dose. The liver enzyme *creatine kinase* is the most commonly used indicator of muscle deterioration, and its level in the blood

> Statin drugs can produce muscle pain and weakness, and severe skeletal muscle disintegration, which may saturate the kidneys and eventually lead to kidney failure.

must be continuously examined in people taking statins. Besides the problems resulting from muscle disintegration, the excess protein from muscle damage in the bloodstream may saturate the kidneys and eventually lead to life-threatening kidney failure.

It has also been shown that statins deplete the body of CoQ_{10}, which is crucial for energy generation in the cell mitochondria and acts as a potent antioxidant. Clearly, CoQ_{10} is extremely important for cardiovascular and heart health, with high levels being found in healthy heart tissue. The heart depends on CoQ_{10} to keep pumping at a rate of 100,000 times per day. By inhibiting the synthesis of the enzyme HMG-CoA reductase (necessary for cholesterol biosynthesis), statins also inhibit the production of CoQ_{10}, as this substance is produced in the same chain of chemical events of cholesterol synthesis.

Another most frequently reported side effects of statin use is negative mental changes, cognitive dysfunction, and transient global amnesia. The brain contains more than 25% of the total cholesterol in the body, and more than 2%

of the brain's total weight is cholesterol. Cholesterol has a critical function in the formation of *synapses* (the connections between neurons). A low cholesterol level affects brain function and also leads to a reduced serotonin level in the brain. Low serotonin levels lead to depression and have been linked to violence and aggression. One well-known NASA physician and former astronaut, *Duane Graveline, M. D.* (see Bibliography), describes in one of his books his experience with transient global amnesia induced by the medication Lipitor® (atorvastatin).

> Statin drugs can induce negative mental behavior, cognitive dysfunction, and transient global amnesia.

There is also evidence that terrible birth defects may occur if an embryo does not get enough cholesterol to develop normally during early pregnancy. Women who know they are pregnant should definitely avoid statins. However, fetal exposure to the drug may happen inadvertently before a woman is even aware she is pregnant. Some clinical trials have shown that statins offer no mortality benefit whatsoever for women, so there seems to be no reason for them to take this drug.

> Fetal exposure to statin drugs can cause birth defects. Pregnant woman should definitely avoid statins.

Cholesterol-lowering medication may also potentially inhibit the synthesis of testosterone and other steroid hormones derived from cholesterol. Some vital functions positively influenced by healthy levels of testosterone are libido, erectile function, cognition, muscle growth, and bone growth.

A staggering amount of evidence seems to indicate that by lowering their cholesterol levels using statin drugs, many people will worsen their physical and mental health and increase their risk of dying prematurely.

To date, the use of statin drugs may be considered a journey into the unknown, and users may think of themselves as part of a mass experiment in progress. Considering the array of negative side effects, on one hand, and the potential cardiovascular health benefits (although small), on the other, it is advisable that statins should be avoided except perhaps for people at high, short-term risk of coronary heart disease, where shortened life expectancy may override concerns of long-term side effects. For people with no signs of coronary heart disease, more judicious preventive measures include a low-to-moderate carbohydrate diet, increased consumption of omega-3 oils, nuts, fresh vegetables and fruits, certain vitanutrient supplements, physical exercise, stress reduction and control, and sound sleep.

> To date, the use of statin drugs may be considered a journey into the unknown, and their use is of considerable risk. However, it seems that people with high-risk of coronary heart disease may benefit from their use.

11.4 GENERAL GUIDELINES FOR A HEALTHY HEART

The following general guidelines may help in the maintenance of a healthy heart.

STRESS. Psychological or chronic stress arouses the release of some hormones (such as the catabolic hormone cortisol, norepinephrine, and epinephrine or adrenaline) that increase heart rate and cause the arteries to spasm and the blood to clot. Stress is one of the primary causes of heart disease. Stress really kills. Do your best to minimize the amount and impact of stress in your life, on a daily basis. Be especially conscious of avoiding stress during and after eating; have your meals in a comfortable and relaxed way, but avoid being inactive (just sitting or sleeping) after a meal.

PHYSICAL EXERCISE. Lack of physical activity results in declining blood sugar control, impaired arterial function, body fat accumulation, and susceptibility to the effects of chronic stress. It is important to exercise regularly. Moderate exercise improves the body antioxidant defense system, builds arterial function and structure, and provides a stimulus for arterial remodeling. Get physical exercises on a regular basis, for at least 30 minutes, on most days of the week.

Be aware that excessive and stressful exercise increases oxidation metabolism and harmful free-radical activity.

SLEEPING HABITS. Poor sleeping habits can be as damaging as chronic stress. Maintain healthy sleeping habits. Get to bed as soon as practical at night, and sleep in a dark, quiet room.

SMOKING. Cigarette smoke is a source of harmful free radicals. Avoid cigarettes, passive (second-hand) smoking, and environmental pollution. Cigarette smoking is pointless and deadly. The combination of stress and cigarette smoking may be fatal.

WEIGHT CONTROL. Maintain a healthy weight, and keep your *body mass index* (BMI) within an adequate range. If you are overweight, start a program of increased activity and calorie restriction to reduce body fat.

BLOOD SUGAR LEVEL. A high blood sugar level, induced by a diet excessively high in carbohydrates (especially those rich in refined carbohydrates and with a high glycemic index), increases free-radical activity, depletes vitamin C, causes excessive blood insulin levels (which may lead to diabetes and obesity), leads to excessive cholesterol levels, and causes increased glycation (oxidation of body proteins). Keep your blood sugar level well within the normal range. Eat a low glycemic load diet; avoid a high-carbohydrate diet and refined and high-GI carbohydrates.

NUTRITION HABITS. Nutritional deficiencies and imbalances, caused by bad eating habits and a deficiency of antioxidants (especially of some important vitamins, minerals, amino acids, plant phenols, carotenoids, and long-chain omega-3 fatty acids), may lead to excessive production of free radicals that directly damage the arteries. Eat fresh meats, poultry, fish, milk derivatives, and eggs, and antioxidant-rich vegetables, fruits, nuts, and seeds to provide potent antioxidants. Skip the low-fat diet fad. Consume long-chain omega-3 lipids such as fish and flaxseed oils regularly. Omega-3 fatty acids have a strong anticoagulant and anti-inflammatory effect (like aspirin) and protect against heart arrhythmias. Enjoy animal and tropical fats in moderation, but avoid refined omega-6 rich vegetable oils and trans fat margarine. Avoid fried foods and processed or packaged foods with a low nutrient-to-calorie ratio, and those containing antinutrient substances. Take antioxidant supplements every day.

ALCOHOL. If you drink alcoholic beverages, consume no more than one or two drinks (beer or a glass of red wine) per day, preferably at meal times, in a pleasant and relaxed environment. Red wine contains phytochemical pigments rich in polyphenols (including resveratrol) and bioflavonoids that exert antioxidant activity and improve blood circulation. Moderate alcohol consumption increases HDL levels and appears to reduce the risk of dying of heart disease by roughly 20%. Heavy or binge drinking seems to have the opposite effect. Avoid excessive alcohol consumption and binge drinking.

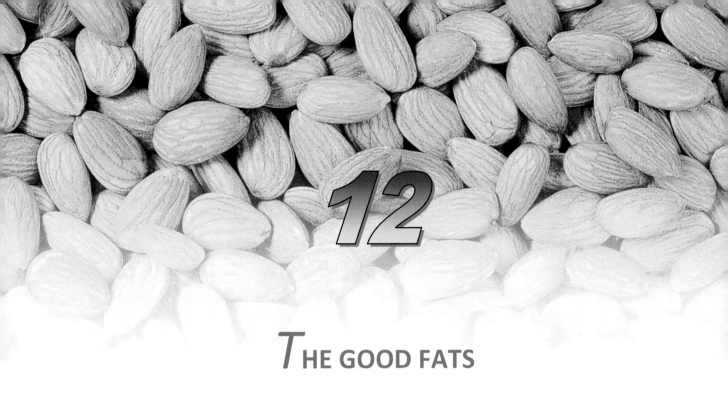

12

THE GOOD FATS

AND OILS

12.1 IMPORTANCE OF HEALTHY FATS AND OILS

*I*n the last few decades, many people avoided eating fats or tried eliminating foods that contain fats from their diet , in an indiscriminate way, erroneously believing that they were improving their health. In the chapters on lipids and cholesterol, it was shown that the various types of lipids are biochemically different. Although some types may be potentially harmful, there are several types of lipids that are essential and play a fundamental role in the maintenance of good health. The term "essential" refers to nutrients that are necessary for good health, but are not synthesized by the body, so they must be obtained from the diet.

The *essential fatty acids* (EFAs) and their derivatives exert important brain functions such as controlling the transmission and reception of pulses between the brain cells and through the nervous system. They regulate other important metabolic processes, including the production of prostaglandins and eicosanoids, which control the cardiovascular system and countless functions in the body. EFAs are like vitamins, and deficiency of EFAs can lead to disease, just like vitamin deficiency. In fact, in the initial studies of EFAs, they were called vitamin F, a term that is now obsolete.

EFA deficiency negatively affects brain function, and can lead to shrinkage in the size and number of brain cells, as well as inhibited communication between them, which can result in problems related to thinking, learning, and growth.

The most dangerous lipids are the following:

➢ (1) Trans fats, the artificial antinutrients present in partially hydrogenated vegetable oils such as margarine, vegetable fats, and industrialized food products that contain these substances (check the labels of industrialized foods).

➢ (2) Refined polyunsaturated vegetable oils that are easily oxidized, such as the industrialized oils of soy, corn, sunflower, and saffron. As a result of refinement, these oils lack antioxidants and natural nutrients, may contain chemical residues, and are packed in inadequate transparent containers that allow the passage of ambient UV light.

➢ (3) Oils heated to high temperatures for long periods (in fried foods), which become highly oxidized and generate cascades of damaging free radicals in the body.

> The essential fatty acids (EFAs) are necessary for good health. They are not synthesized by the body and must be obtained from the diet.

Research continues to show that saturated fat is not intrinsically harmful. However, it may potentially become harmful when consumed in excess and as part of an unbalanced diet that is deficient in antioxidant vitanutrients, rich in sugars and refined glycemic carbohydrates, and contains oxidizing substances that generate free radicals.

According to specialists, the ingestion of fat must be selective, and the healthy ones should contribute to about 30% of daily calories. To avoid storing body fat, total ingested calories should be less than (or equal to) the total of expended calories. It is important to maintain a good balance between omega-6 and omega-3 fatty acids (avoiding excessive consumption of omega-6 oils) and to ingest adequate quantities of complete proteins, soluble fibers, and vitanutrients such as vitamins, minerals, and antioxidants. Many vitamins (such as A, D, E, and K, which are fat soluble) and antioxidants (such as beta-carotene and lycopene, also fat soluble) are adequately absorbed by the body only when ingested with fatty foods.

12.2 FISH OIL

*M*any important studies have shown that people who eat fish regularly are healthier than those who don't. Seafood and cold-water fatty fish (such as sardines, mackerel, salmon, tuna, and anchovy) are rich in omega-3 fatty acids. Fish oil is an effective anticlotting agent. It protects the arteries, thins the blood, and reduces blood coagulation that promotes infarct and heart attacks.

The benefits of omega-3 fatty acids for the heart and for protection against cardiovascular diseases are well documented in nutrition literature. They reduce blood levels of triglycerides and LDL (bad cholesterol), prevent the formation of fatty deposits in the arteries, act as anticlotting agents to prevent blood clot formation, prevent strokes, lower blood pressure, and protect against fatal heart spasms. They recover the elasticity of the arteries and maintain them. There is evidence of the benefits of fish oil in the prevention of breast and colon cancer as well as in protecting the lungs of cigarette smokers.

> The ingestion of fats must be selective, and the healthy ones should contribute to about 30% of the daily ingested calories.

The benefits of omega-3 fatty acids go well beyond protection to the cardiovascular system and cancer prevention. Fish oil is a valuable treatment for rheumatism, arthritis, and other inflammatory diseases, skin problems (such as eczema and psoriasis), inflammatory diseases of the colon, kidney diseases, depression, and auto-immune diseases such as multiple sclerosis, scleroderma, and lupus. Fish oil helps to prevent osteoporosis by inhibiting the production of a prostaglandin that limits bone growth. It also enhances the activity of the insulin-like growth factor IGF-1, a substance closely related to the *human growth hormone* (HGH), which is presently considered of great relevance to slow down the aging process.

Fish oils are rich in the fatty acids *eicosapentaenoic* (EPA) and *docosahexaenoic* (DHA). They are long-chain polyunsaturated fatty acids of the omega-3 family. EPA has 20 carbon atoms in its molecular chain, with five double bonds, whereas DHA has 22 carbon atoms in its molecular chain, with six double bonds.

EPA and DHA are also found in commercial capsules that contain omega-3 oils extracted from fish and with relatively low concentrations of vitamins A and D. Oil supplements extracted from fish liver are not recommended due to their high concentrations of vitamins A and D, which may be toxic if consumed in excess for long periods.

> Fish oil provides countless benefits to our health, including protection to the cardiovascular system and anti-inflammatory effects.

The benefits of adding fish to the diet are numerous. Eating fish (preferably not fried) two to three times a week, especially cold-water fatty fish such as sardines, salmon, mackerel, herring, anchovy, tuna, and trout, can reduce the chances of heart disease or cancer.

Table 12.1 shows the EPA and DHA content of some sea foods, whereas Table 12.2 shows the amount of omega-3 oils and total lipids contained in these foods. The quantities given in the tables represent average values.

Dietary supplements of omega-3 oils extracted from fish are recommended by many nutrition experts, even if fish is a normal part of the diet, for complementary reasons. One to three grams per day are suggested. Gelatin capsules of omega-3 fish oils are common in the market, and each 1g capsule usually contains 180mg of EPA and 120mg of DHA.

TABLE 12.1 – EPA and DHA content of selected sea foods.

FOOD (100g)	EPA + DHA (g)	FAT (g)	CHOLESTEROL (mg)	CALORIES (cal)
Sardines	1.0 – 1.4	11	70	200
Salmon	1.0 – 1.4	7	75	200
Trout	0.5	4	55	150
Crab	0.4	1.5	80	120
Tuna	0.3	5	30	150
Shrimp	0.2	1.5	130	110
Flounder	0.2	1	45	120
Lobster	0.2	1	95	120
Cod	0.2	1	35	100

12.3 OLIVE OIL

Extra virgin olive oil is sometimes called the "green gold of the Mediterranean". Scientific research has confirmed what has been believed since ancient times: *extra virgin olive oil* is of great importance for the prevention and treatment of cardiovascular diseases, some forms of cancer, and inflammatory conditions such as arthritis. It is also necessary for normal cellular function.

To obtain all the benefits from olive oil, it must be virgin or unrefined. Three forms of olive oil are normally found in the market. The extra virgin olive oil comes from the first cold pressing of selected olives, while virgin olive oil also comes from cold pressing but from nonselected olives. Normal pure olive oil is produced by pressing and heating the mass generated from the first cold pressing. In general, cold-pressed virgin oils are better than those extracted by heating or using chemical substances.

> It is recommended the ingestion of one to three grams per day of omega-3 oils, which contain EPA and DHA.

FOOD (100g)	OMEGA-3 (g)	TOTAL FAT (g)
Sardines	3	10 - 12
Mackerel	2 - 3	9 - 14
Salmon	1 - 2	5 - 9
Tuna	1 - 2	4 - 7
Trout	1 - 2	4 - 5
Herring	1 - 2	6 - 9
Sablefish	1.5	13
Anchovy	1.5	6.5
Mullet	1	4.5
Halibut	0.5 - 1	2
Pompano	0.5	9
Catfish	0.5	3.5
Perch	0.5	2.5
Bass	0.5	2
Hake	0.5	2.5
Shark	0.5	2
Oyster	0.5	2.5
Crab	0.5	1.5
Shrimp	0.5	1 – 1.5
Flounder	0.3	1
Swordfish	0.2	2
Cod	0.2	1

TABLE 12.2 – Content of omega-3 and total fat in selected sea foods.

Olive oil consists mostly of *oleic acid*, a monounsaturated fatty acid (MUFA) of the omega-9 family, but it also includes smaller quantities of the polyunsaturated fatty acids (PUFAs) *linoleic* (LA), of the omega-6 family, and *alpha-linolenic* (LNA), of the omega-3 family. It also contains *palmitoleic acid*, of the omega-7 family, and saturated fats of vegetable origin (*palmitic* and *stearic fatty acids*), as shown in Table 12.3. Olive oil also contains several important minor components including antioxidants such as beta-carotene, tocopherols of the vitamin E family, phytosterols (such as beta-sistosterol), and chlorophylls rich in magnesium.

Extra virgin olive oil is stable and not easily oxidized, even when slightly heated, providing beneficial effects to the cardiovascular system. It increases the blood levels of the high-density lipoprotein (HDL, good cholesterol) and protects cholesterol from oxidation. It also diminishes the adhesion tendency of the blood platelets, thus preventing formation of blood clots.

Extra virgin olive oil increases the blood levels of HDL (good cholesterol) and plays an important role in the prevention and treatment of cardiovascular disease and inflammatory conditions.

TABLE 12.3 - Content of fatty acids in olive oil.

FATTY ACID	PERCENTAGE
Oleic acid - MUFA - omega-9	63 - 83
Linoleic acid (LA) - omega-6	3.5 - 20
Alpha-linolenic acid (LNA) - omega-3	0.1 - 6
Palmitoleic acid - omega-7	0.5 - 3
Saturated vegetable fat - SFA	7.5 - 18

12.4 FLAXSEED (LINSEED)

*F*laxseed oil constitutes one of the richest sources of omega-3 fatty acids, particularly of the essential triunsaturated *alpha-linolenic acid* (LNA). Flaxseed oil also contains monounsaturated fatty acids (*oleic acid*), polyunsaturated fatty acids of the omega-6 family, such as the essential diunsaturated *linoleic acid* (LA), and saturated fatty acids of vegetable origin, as shown in Table 12.4.

We are not referring to the flaxseed oil that is commercially used in paints, dyes, and varnishes (these are not meant for human use) but to the delicate organic oil extracted from flaxseed through a careful cold-pressing process. Because flaxseed oil is a delicate and perishable product, it must be adequately protected during processing, handling, and storage. The benefits of the oil remain only if it is kept fresh and in its natural state. The flaxseeds must be cold-pressed (below 40°C), and the oil must be unrefined, nonfiltered, nondeodorized, and kept refrigerated in opaque containers.

The best way to obtain the benefits of flaxseed oil, however, is through the ingestion of flaxseeds recently ground. The human digestive system is unable to break down whole flaxseeds, which pass through undigested. Grinding them is the way to release the many nutrients so that they can be absorbed by the body. A coffee grinder can be used to grind the flaxseeds. The powder must be stored in an opaque container and kept refrigerated. You can then mix it with foods such as yogurt, salad, and fruit.

TABLE 12.4 – Content of main fatty acids in the fatty part of flaxseeds.

FATTY ACID	PERCENTAGE
Alpha-linolenic acid (LNA) - omega-3	57
Oleic acid - MUFA - omega-9	18
Linoleic acid (LA) - omega-6	16
Saturated vegetable fat - SFA	9

Besides the oil, flaxseeds are also rich in soluble fibers that aid in reducing blood glucose and cholesterol levels, and they are particularly rich in *lignans*, which are *phytohormonal* or *phytoestrogen* fibers. Phytoestrogens are estrogen-like chemicals that also act as antioxidants. They can normalize estrogen metabolism in women, removing excess estrogen that may promote breast cancer. There are two major types of phytoestrogens: *isoflavones* (present in soybeans) and lignans. They mimic the effects of the hormone estrogen and compete with a woman's endogenous estrogen. The phytoestrogens bind to estrogen receptors in the body, thereby blocking the stronger, cancer-stimulating estrogen. Many studies have shown that the anti-estrogen lignans of flaxseeds also reduce the influence of other hormones on premenstrual stress, and they help to prevent breast cancer, colon cancer, and other cancers of hormonal origin. They also decrease prostate cancer cell proliferation. Because of the powerful antioxidant and anti-inflammatory properties of lignans, they also help protect the heart.

One portion of 100g of flaxseed contains about 23g of total fat (which contain a valuable 13g of LNA), 19g of proteins, 27g of carbohydrates, and 21g of soluble fiber, providing a total of about 390 calories. Flaxseed also contains significant levels of minerals such as calcium, magnesium, manganese, and potassium, as well as vitamin E and beta-carotene.

> Flaxseed is rich in oils of the omega-3 family, essential fatty acids, and soluble fibers.

Countless scientific studies have demonstrated the beneficial effects of flaxseed, which aids in disease prevention and reduction. These include the following:

➢ Increased blood levels of HDL.
➢ Decreased blood levels of LDL.
➢ Normalized blood pressure.
➢ Reduced circulatory problems.
➢ Increased burning of body fat.
➢ Relief from depression, fatigue, and allergies.
➢ Cure of skin disorders such as acne, psoriasis, eczema, and dryness.
➢ Prevention of breast cancer.
➢ Prevention of diabetes.
➢ Improvement of problems related to mental health.
➢ Slowed aging process.

12.5 PRIMROSE AND BORAGE OILS

*O*il extracted from the seeds of the primrose (an early-flowering perennial plant with pale yellow flowers) is rich in *gamma-linolenic acid* (GLA), a nonessential fatty acid of the omega-6 family. The oils from the seeds of borage (a coarse, hairy, blue-flowered herb) and blackcurrant (a bush that bears this edible soft fruit) also constitute good sources of GLA. The only known source of GLA from animal origin is breast milk, which contains about 0.25 to 1% of GLA in healthy mothers.

GLA is a rare nutrient that can alleviate many health problems such as heart disease, arthritis, and skin disorders, among others. GLA is of fundamental importance for the production of prostaglandins (PGs), particularly of the family designated by the subscript 1 (see the chapter on fatty acids and health). PGs are substances similar to hormones, but of short reach and duration, that control important functions in all organs of the body. PGE_1, produced from GLA, exerts beneficial functions in the control of cardiovascular diseases, cancer, arthritis, allergies, asthma, and autoimmune diseases, and it slows aging. It modulates feminine hormones and influences the release of brain neurotransmitters such as epinephrine, norepinephrine, dopamine, and serotonin (produced from the essential amino acid tryptophan).

> Primrose oil is a source of gamma-linolenic acid (GLA), which is of fundamental importance for the production of prostaglandins (PGs).

GLA exerts a stimulating effect in brown fat tissue, producing some prostaglandins that accelerate mitochondria activity in these tissues, thus helping to reduce body fat and weight. It also helps in the production of high-energy *adenosine triphosphate* (ATP) molecules, which provide energy for muscular activity. GLA also exerts a beneficial effect on the skin, making it flexible and soft.

Although the body can produce GLA from the essential linoleic acid (LA), many people do not synthesize enough GLA for various reasons, which results in health problems. For the production of GLA, starting from LA (in the cis form), the body needs vitamin B_6, zinc, and magnesium (see Figure 8.1 in the chapter on fatty acids and health). These substances are necessary for the production of the enzyme delta-6-desaturase (D6D), which allows LA to convert into GLA. However, many factors act as blockers, including the presence of LA in the trans form, excess saturated fats, high blood cholesterol, excess alcohol, radiation, presence of carcinogenic substances, and advanced age. To guarantee optimum levels of PGs, it is important to fortify the production of GLA by eating adequate amounts of EFAs, as well as consuming GLA directly (it is available in nutritional supplements from natural sources). Deficiency of EFAs leads to early aging, mental problems, cardiovascular disturbances, arterial hypertension, and many other unhealthy metabolic issues.

Primrose oil contains about 9% of GLA and about 70% of LA. The oil from borage seeds contains higher amounts of GLA (about three times more). Because these plant seeds are not normally part of human diets, nutritional supplements may be necessary. Normally, one gel capsule of 500mg of

> Deficiency of EFAs leads to early aging, mental problems, cardiovascular disturbances, and arterial hypertension.

commercially available primrose oil contains about 45mg of GLA, whereas one gel capsule of 1,000mg of borage oil contains about 240mg. Therefore, borage oil is a more practical and economical source of GLA. Preference must be given to supplements that contain oils extracted without the use of heat (cold pressing), which protects the delicate chemical structure of the oils. Two to three capsules per day are normally recommended following the orientation of a nutritionist or a health specialist. Nutritional complementation of GLA is important for women during pregnancy and breast feeding. GLA is also recommended to reduce colic and premenstrual stress.

Primrose and borage oils provide countless health benefits that are well documented in nutritional literature:

- ➤ Relieve pain, colic, and premenstrual stress.
- ➤ Combat rheumatoid arthritis, in moderate cases.
- ➤ Avoid benign breast alterations.
- ➤ Reduce weight in overweight people.
- ➤ Reduce blood cholesterol.
- ➤ Normalize blood pressure.
- ➤ Aid in preventing coronary problems.
- ➤ Slow the progress of multiple sclerosis.
- ➤ Heal or improve eczema.
- ➤ Help maintain a healthy skin.
- ➤ Improve acne, when taken with zinc.
- ➤ Improve fingernail growth.
- ➤ Normalize saliva and tear production.
- ➤ Help repair nerve damage caused by diabetes.
- ➤ Improve behavior of hyperactive children.
- ➤ Normalize emotional problems (aggression, irritability, anxiety, and nervousness).
- ➤ Alleviate hangover.
- ➤ Help repair liver tissue damaged by alcohol abuse.

12.6 LECITHIN

Lecithin, also known as *phosphatidyl-choline*, is a lipid that belongs to the class of *phospholipids*, which are lipids that have the mineral phosphorus in their molecule. Like triglycerides, they are also structured in the glycerol molecule, but they have two fatty acid molecules (which may be saturated or unsaturated) and a residue of phosphatidyl-choline chemically bound each to the glycerol molecule.

Lecithin is fundamental to life and aids in forming cell membranes. It is an essential protector of each cell, especially of the nervous system. Lecithin contributes to the production of *acetyl-choline*, an important neurotransmitter involved in muscular contraction. It is not an essential lipid, because it can be synthesized by the liver starting from choline. Foods such as egg yolks, soybeans, and peanuts have high concentrations of choline and phosphatidyl-choline. The body digests (decomposes) lecithin taken in through foods or food supplements before it is absorbed (the liver synthesizes all the lecithin finally used by the body).

Lecithin is a natural *emulsifier* of fats. It can break or liquefy the fat present in the blood vessels, and it helps to maintain the fluidity of cholesterol and triglycerides in the blood and in other fluids, thereby preventing plaque accumulation on artery walls. Studies have shown that lecithin protects the arteries from damage that may result from excessive blood cholesterol. It also helps to reduce arterial blood pressure, promoting the relaxation of blood vessels and improving blood flow.

> Lecithin is a phospholipid that aids in forming cell membranes, especially of the nervous system, and in producing important neurotransmitters.

Lecithin also plays an important role in the production of neurotransmitters, involved in the transmission of chemical signals to the brain, thereby influencing emotional and physical behavior, and improving memory. It is responsible for the overall functioning of the brain and nervous system. Lecithin is present in all living cells and is found amply diffused in the tissues of animals and plants.

Lecithin extracted from soybeans is normally used in dietary supplements, and it consists of a mixture of three phospholipids dissolved in soy oil, used as medium. These supplements are found commercially in three forms: granular, capsule, and liquid (or paste) form. Gel capsules with 1,200mg of lecithin extracted from soybeans are common in the market.

Other substances associated with lecithin are *choline* and *inositol*. These nutrients exert functions closely related to the vitamin B complex although they do not belong to the vitamin B group, and they function as coenzymes in body metabolism.

Choline is necessary for the production of the neurotransmitter acetyl-choline, and it is considered a useful tonic for the brain that improves memory and learning. It is essential for the health of the myelin sheath that surrounds the nerves, which constitutes a main component of the nerve fibers, and it plays an important role in the transmission of nerve impulses. It is also involved in the use of fats and cholesterol by the body. Choline combines chemically with fatty acids and phosphoric acid in the liver, forming lecithin, and it is fundamental for the health of the liver and kidneys. The best source of choline is lecithin, which is found in egg yolks, liver, brewer's yeast, soybeans, peanuts, and wheat germ. Choline is synthesized in the liver through the chemical interaction between folic acid, vitamin B_{12}, and the amino acid *methionine*.

The amount of choline needed daily is not established, but it is estimated to be around 1g or more. Deficiency can cause high blood pressure, cirrhosis, formation of fatty deposits in the liver, liver degeneration, and atherosclerosis. It is also believed that Alzheimer's disease may be caused partly by deficiency of acetyl-choline in the brain.

Inositol plays a role similar to choline in the transport of fats from the liver to the cells, helping in fat metabolism, reducing blood cholesterol, preventing atherosclerosis, nourishing brain cells and the nervous system, and protecting the liver, kidneys, and heart. Similar to choline, it is found in the tissues of animals and plants, and the best source is lecithin.

Inositol, choline, vitamin B_{12}, and methionine are linked to the processing of fats in the liver and are usually called *lipotropic* nutrients or fat-burners. This group of nutrients supports and protects liver function and enhances the liver's ability to metabolize hormones such as estrogen. The lipotropic nutrients are also beneficial for reducing the risk of cancer related to hormones in women and in reducing premenstrual stress. Pills containing lipotropic nutrients are normally available in the

> The lipotropic nutrients (inositol, choline, vitamin B_{12}, and methionine) support liver function.

pharmaceutical commerce under several brand names.

12.7 NUTS AND SEEDS

*T*he high calorie content of nuts and seeds may cause wariness in some people, but if we look only at the fat and calorie content of foods, we may lose sight of their effects in body metabolism and hormonal balance.

In general, nuts and seeds are rich in good-quality, beneficial fats, mainly MUFAs, which reduce LDL and increase HDL. They are also rich in protein, vitamin E, fiber, and important minerals. However, due to their high calorie content, it is wise to ration them within the daily limit of calories set by your level of exercise or ability to burn calories.

Nuts and seeds have high nutritional values, compared to other foods that are rich in refined carbohydrates. For example, 70g of nuts provides about 400 calories with a high nutritional density, whereas 100g of cookies made of refined flour and sugar also provides 400 calories, but with no nutritional value (empty calories). More important than their calorie content are the hormonal reactions they stimulate in the body.

Nuts and seeds aid in the stabilization of blood levels of glucose and insulin, lower blood cholesterol levels, normalize blood pressure, provide nutrients and essential fats for prostaglandin synthesis (which stimulate weight loss), and promote satiety ("full" feeling). On the other hand, foods such as cookies and biscuits (without fat) have fewer calories than nuts and seeds, but their content of sugar and refined flour increases blood levels of glucose, insulin, triglycerides, and cholesterol, causes harmful fluctuations in the blood glucose levels, increases hunger for more carbohydrates, and impairs the production of prostaglandins. High blood levels of insulin and unbalanced prostaglandins promote obesity.

> Nuts and seeds are foods of high nutritional density and rich in beneficial lipids.

In their natural state, nuts such as pecans, almonds, hazelnuts, pistachios, cashew, Brazil, and macadamias, are dense in nutrients, rich in essential fatty acids, proteins, soluble fibers, vitamin E, folic acid, and they provide important minerals such as calcium, phosphorus, magnesium, zinc, selenium, and potassium, as well as some important phytonutrients. Brazil nuts, for example, grown in the rich soil of the Amazon region, are rich in selenium, a powerful antioxidant and anticarcinogenic substance. One single Brazil nut may provide about 25µg to 50µg of selenium (the same amount in a commercial selenium pill). Macadamias are extremely rich in monounsaturated fatty acids (like those found in olive oil) and vitamins of the B complex.

> Avoid consuming nuts and seeds toasted with hydrogenated vegetable oils (vegetable fat).

Nuts are also rich in the amino acid *arginine*, necessary for the production of *nitric oxide* (NO), which helps to relax blood vessels and thus facilitates blood flow. They also make the blood platelets less sticky and therefore less likely to form clots in the arteries.

Seeds such as sesame, sunflower, pumpkin, chia, and flaxseeds are also dense in nutrients. The statement "good things come in small packets" certainly applies here. As shown previously in this chapter, flaxseeds are good sources of essential omega-3 fatty acids (as alpha-linolenic acid, LNA), soluble fibers (lignans), and other important vitanutrients.

Table 12.5 shows the relative concentrations of some important minerals present in selected nuts and seeds. Table 8.1 (in the chapter on fatty acids and health) shows the relative proportion of macronutrients (carbohydrates, proteins, and lipids) and calories in these foods.

To best enjoy the many healthy properties of nuts and seeds, it is important that they were organically grown in mineral-rich soils, are fresh (close to their natural state), are kept refrigerated, and, if possible, are unshelled just before eating. They should not be excessively toasted (at most, slightly toasted) and certainly not fried or toasted with hydrogenated vegetable oils (vegetable fat). Heating to high temperatures transforms part of their beneficial oils into harmful substances, destroying some fatty acids and vitamins. Nuts and seeds with sugar coats or coatings made with refined flour and hydrogenated vegetable oils should be avoided. Check the labels of industrialized nuts to determine that they were not toasted with vegetable fat.

TABLE 12.5 – Relative concentrations (in mg) of some important minerals present in selected nuts, seeds, and legumes.

FOOD (100g)	Ca	P	Mg	K	Zn	Cu
Almonds	280	555	305	780	5.0	1.1
Brazil nuts	180	605	230	605	46	1.8
Cashew nuts	45	495	265	570	5.7	2.3
Hazel nuts	80	430	185	520	3.2	1.3
Macadamias	70	140	120	370	1.8	0.3
Peanuts	55	355	175	655	3.2	0.7
Pecans	35	295	130	395	5.7	1.2
Pistachios	135	510	160	1105	1.4	1.2
Pumpkin seeds	45	1190	545	820	7.5	1.4
Sesame seeds	130	785	350	410	10.4	
Soybeans (dried)	270	650	230	1365	4.8	1.1
Sunflower seeds	120	715	355	700	5.0	1.8

Note: **Ca** = Calcium; **P** = Phosphorus; **Mg** = Magnesium; **K** = Potassium; **Zn** = Zinc; **Cu** = Copper.

Although peanuts belong to the legume family, they have characteristics similar to nuts and seeds from a nutritional point of view. They are also nutritionally dense, with many positive properties, and rich in monounsaturated fatty acids and minerals. They also contain carbohydrates of low GI and are good sources of protein. However, when consuming peanuts, research whether they were adequately stored to prevent the proliferation of a fungus called *aflatoxin*. This fungus is potentially carcinogenic and easily grows in this type of

> Peanuts belong to the legume family, but have nutritional properties similar to nuts and seeds.

legume, as well as in corn. According to current research, it is believed that this substance is responsible for thousands of cases of liver cancer, annually, in the United States.

Many recent studies have shown that nuts and seeds can significantly reduce the incidence of cardiovascular disease. Due to their high caloric value, the principle of "quality over quantity" must be applied here. Therefore, it is recommended to ration these foods within the daily limit of calories set by your ability to burn calories and maintain an optimum weight.

GLOSSARY

Acetyl-Coenzyme A (Acetyl-CoA). Substance involved in many biochemical reactions and formed in an intermediate step of the oxidation cycle (burning) of cell organic fuels, mainly carbohydrates and fats. It is also the substrate for acetylcholine and cholesterol biosynthesis. It consists of a two-carbon acetate group linked to coenzyme A.

Acetylcholine. One of the many chemical neurotransmitters in both the peripheral nervous system and the central nervous system.

Acidosis. Increased acidity of the blood plasma that results from an inadequate metabolism. It occurs when the arterial blood pH (normally between 7.35 and 7.45; slightly alkaline) falls below 7.35.

Adenosine Triphosphate (ATP). High-energy molecule formed in the metabolism of cellular fuels and provides energy in muscular contractions. It constitutes an energy currency in the processes that involve energy exchange within the body.

Adipose Tissue. Fatty cells distributed through the body's tissues. Scientific name for body fat. It is one of the main types of connective tissues.

AGEs. Advanced glycation end-products. They result from a chain of chemical reactions after an initial glycation reaction. They are formed from sugars and are considered to be a factor in aging and some age-related diseases.

Aldose. A simple sugar (monosaccharide) that contains only one aldehyde radical (- CH=O) in its molecule.

Alimentary Calorie. Thermal energy, used in nutrition, equivalent to one thousand physical calories (1,000cal or 1kcal). See also calorie.

Alpha-Linolenic Acid (LNA). Essential fatty acid (octadecatrienoic), of the omega-3 family, present in many vegetable oils. It consists of an 18-carbon chain carboxylic acid with three cis double bonds that occur in the carbons 3, 6, and 9, counting from the methyl radical (- CH_3).

Alzheimer's Disease. Degenerative disease of the brain that leads to a form of dementia. Characterized by accumulation of plaques in certain regions of the brain and degeneration of a certain class of neurons.

Amine Group. Chemical radical in the form (- NH_2), or (- NHR), or (- NR_2), as part of an organic molecule, where R denotes an alkyl group.

Amino Acid. Elementary building block of proteins, composed basically of a carboxylic acid radical (- COOH) and an amine radical (- NH2), bonded to a chain of carbon atoms that is specific to each amino acid.

Amphiphilic Substance. A chemical substance that possesses both hydrophilic (polar, water-soluble) and lipophilic (non-polar, fat-soluble) properties. Also called amphipathic substance.

Amylopectin. Carbohydrate (polysaccharide) that consists of highly branched polymers of interconnected D-glucose units. Amylopectin and amylose constitute the two components of starch.

Amylose. Carbohydrate (polysaccharide) that consists of linear polymers of interconnected D-glucose units.

Anabolism. Set of metabolic reactions that absorb energy, in which complex biological molecules are synthesized in the body from simpler components. Many anabolic processes are powered by adenosine triphosphate (ATP).

Androgen. Generic term relative to factors that originate the male characteristics.

Androsterone. Male steroid hormone with weak androgenic activity. It is less active than testosterone.

Aneurysm. A localized, blood-filled balloon-like bulge in the wall of a blood vessel. Aneurysms can commonly occur in arteries at the base of the brain.

Antibody. Large y-shaped protein produced by the immune system to identify and neutralize foreign elements (antigen) introduced in the body, such as bacteria and viruses. Also known as immunoglobulin.

Antigen. Foreign and potentially harmful invader in the body that causes the immune system to produce antibodies against it.

Antioxidant. Natural or synthetic substance (including vitamins and minerals) capable of inhibiting the oxidation of other molecules. They are able to provide electrons to neutralize free radicals and oxygen derivatives that can induce degenerative oxidation in fatty acids and cells in the body.

Apoenzyme. Inactive enzyme due to absence of a cofactor.

Apolipoprotein. Protein component of a blood lipoprotein, also called apoprotein. It binds to lipids, such as fat and cholesterol, to form blood lipoproteins that transport lipids through the lymphatic and circulatory system.

Arachidonic Acid (AA). Essential fatty acid (eicosatetraenoic), of the omega-6 family, formed of a 20-carbon chain with four cis double bonds that occur in the carbons 6, 9, 12, and 15, counting from the methyl radical (- CH_3).

Arterial Hypertension. High blood pressure in the arteries.

Arterial Plaque. See atheroma.

Atherogenic. Substances or processes that can cause the development of atherosclerosis.

Atheroma. Plaque of fatty and fibrous substances, made up mostly of macrophage cells (debris), fatty substances, calcium, and fibrous connectice tissues, that accumulate in artery walls (with swelling), and leads to atherosclerosis (a chronic inflammatory disease of the blood vessels).

Atherosclerosis. A chronic inflammatory disease characterized by the formation and accumulation of multiple plaques of fatty and fibrous substances in the wall of blood vessels, that cause thickening and elasticity loss of artery walls. The narrowing and hardening of blood vessels cause a gradual blockage of blood flow and may eventually stop it, leading to death of tissues fed by the artery. Also known as arteriosclerotic vascular disease (ASVD).

ATP. See adenosine triphosphate.

Autoimmune Disease. Disease in which the body's immune system loses part of its auto-tolerance and produces antibodies against substances and tissues normally present in the body. The body's uncontrolled immune system attacks its own cells.

Bacteria. A large domain of prokaryotic microorganisms having a few micrometers in length. They are present in most habitats on Earth, in organic matter, and the live bodies of plants and animals.

Beta-carotene. Red-orange pigment, abundant in plants and fruits (mainly carrots), that exerts antioxidant action. It helps to protect the body against free radical activity and is a precursor (inactive form) to vitamin A.

Bile Acids. Steroid acids derived from cholesterol, made in the liver and stored in the gallbladder. They are secreted into the intestine (duodenum) and act as an emulsifier of dietary lipids to promote digestion and absorption of fatty acids. Also called bile or gall, a bitter-tasting dark-green to yellowish-brown fluid.

Bile Salts. Bile acid compounds with a cation, usually sodium. See also bile acids.

Bioflavonoids. Phytochemical substances, present in plants and fruits, that exert protective antioxidant activity in the body. They are the most important plant pigments for flower coloration producing yellow or red/blue pigmentation in petals.

Brown Adipose Tissue. Special adipose tissue rich in mitochondria (which make it brown) located mainly in the upper chest, behind the neck, and along the spine, that helps in the production of heat energy (thermogenesis) from extra food calories.

Brown Fat. See brown adipose tissue.

Calorie (cal). Thermal energy necessary to raise the temperature of one gram of water from $14.5°C$ to $15.5°C$, at normal atmospheric pressure. See also alimentary calorie.

Calorie Restriction. A dietary regimen that restricts calorie intake, without malnutrition, presently believed to improve age-related health and to slow the aging process.

Cancer. Broad group of various diseases that involve abnormal cell growth. They are caused by cell DNA damage that leads to cell mutation, giving rise to uncontrolled cell reproduction. Cancer may spread to other parts of the body (metastasis) through the lymphatic system or bloodstream.

Carbohydrate. Organic compound that has the general chemical formula $C_n(H_2O)_m$ where n and m represent integer numbers greater than (or equal to) three. Also called saccharide or polysaccharide (from the Greek word *sákkharon*, which means *sugar*).

Carbonyl Group. Chemical radical or functional group ($=C=O$) as part of an organic molecule.

Carboxyl Group. Chemical radical or functional group (- COOH) as part of an organic molecule.

Carcinogen. Any substance or agent (as radiation) that damages cell DNA, leading to cellular mutation and uncontrolled cellular reproduction (cancer).

Cardiac Sphincter. Circular muscle or anatomical ring valve that controls the opening and closure between the esophagus and the stomach. Also termed cardia (lower esophageal sphincter).

Carotenenoids. Organic pigments present in plants and colored vegetables that strengthen the immune system and exert protective antioxidant action in the body. They are classified as xanthophylls (which contain oxygen) and carotenes (without oxygen).

Catabolism. Set of biochemical reactions that break down nutrients, cell elements, and molecules into smaller units (metabolic degradation) and release energy.

Catalyst. Substance that promotes or accelerates a chemical reaction and that is not consumed by the reaction itself.

Cell Membrane. Biological double layer of fatty substances (phospholipids) with embedded proteins, that surrounds each cell. This membrane protects the cells from the outside surroundings.

Cerebrovascular Accident (CVA). See stroke.

Chiral Center. Molecule stereocenter that consists of an atom holding a set of groups of atoms in a spatial arrangement which is not superposable on its mirror image. An interchanging of any two groups leads to a stereoisomer. Also called asymmetric center.

Cholesterol. Organic chemical substance of the steroid (lipid) class, necessary for human health, produced by the liver or ingested from animal sources. It is an essential component of cell membranes. Excessive levels of cholesterol in the blood have been linked to cardiovascular disease, when damaged by oxidative reactions.

Choline. Essential water-soluble nutrient, usually grouped within the B-complex vitamins, involved in many nervous functions and lipid metabolism. It is a precursor molecule for the neurotransmitter acetylcholine. Lecithin, which is rich in phosphatidylcholine, is also a good source of choline.

Chromosome. Organized structure of a protein complex, RNA, and one single coiled DNA molecule, that constitutes part or all of a body's genome.

Chylomicron. Lipoprotein particle present in the blood that transports lipids (mainly triglycerides), absorbed from the intestines after food digestion, to other locations in the body.

Citric Acid Cycle. Series of biochemical reactions, promoted by enzymes, that occur in aerobic organisms to generate energy through the oxidation of acetate derived from carbohydrates, fats, and proteins, releasing carbon dioxide and water. Also known as Krebs cycle or tricarboxylic acid cycle (TCA cycle).

Cloning. Biological reproduction of similar copies of a cell DNA segment, to produce populations of genetically identical individuals.

Coenzyme. Organic molecule essential for the catalytic activity of an enzyme.

Coenzyme Q$_{10}$. Vitamin-like (oil-soluble) substance, present in most eukaryotic cells (primarily in the mitochondria). It is essential for energy production within the cells, including the heart muscle cells. Also known as ubiquinone.

Cofactor. Organic or inorganic molecule (non-protein chemical compound), or metallic ion, that is necessary for the catalytic activity of an enzyme. An inactive enzyme, without the cofactor, is called an apoenzyme.

Cold-Pressed. Term used in the extraction of oils from some vegetables by compression, without the use of heat or chemical solvents.

Complete Protein. Food rich in proteins that contains all the nine essential amino acids in appropriate proportions for body consumption and anabolism.

CVA (Cerebrovascular Accident). See stroke.

Cytoplasm. Gel-like substance that holds all the contents or sub-structures (organelles) of a cell, excluding the membrane and nucleus.

Dalton (D). A mass unit that corresponds to 1/12 of the mass of the carbon atom isotope 12.

Dehydroepiandrosterone (DHEA). A 19-carbon endogenous steroid hormone also known as mother-hormone. It is a precursor for more than forty other important adrenal hormones, including all the adrenal steroids, such as cortisol (stress hormone) and the sexual hormones (progesterone, estrogen, and testosterone).

Deoxyribonucleic Acid (DNA). Polymer of deoxynucleotides, a nucleic acid, whose sequence of segments (genes) codify the genetic instructions for the development and functioning of living cells and organisms.

DHA. See docosahexaenoic acid..

DHEA. Sea dehydroepiandrosterone.

Diabetes Mellitus Type 1. Disease characterized by insufficient production of insulin by the pancreas, associated with a damaged pancreas. The lack of insulin leads to increased blood and urine glucose.

Diabetes Mellitus Type 2. Disease characterized by excessive production of insulin (hyperinsulinism), stressing the pancreas. It is associated with excessive blood glucose levels and cell insulin resistance. Also known as adult-onset diabetes.

Disaccharides. Carbohydrates (sugars) that consist of two monosaccharide molecules (single sugars) joined by a covalent glycosidic bond. Common examples in nutrition are sucrose (table sugar), lactose, and maltose.

DNA. See deoxyribonucleic acid.

Docosahexaenoic Acid (DHA). Essential fatty acid, of the omega-3 family, formed of a 22-carbon chain with six cis double bonds that occur in the carbons 3, 6, 9 12, 15, and 18, counting from the methyl radical ($- CH_3$). Main source is fish oil.

Duodenum. First section (upper part) of the small intestine.

EFA. See essential fatty acids.

Eicosanoids. Chemical compounds derived from arachidonic acid (AA) with twenty carbon atoms in their molecule. They exert complex control over many bodily systems, including inflammation processes. They are classified in four families: prostaglandins, prostacyclins, thromboxanes, and leukotrienes.

Eicosapentaenoic Acid (EPA). Essential fatty acid, of the omega-3 family, formed of a 20-carbon chain with five cis double bonds that occur in the carbons 3, 6, 9 12, and 15, counting from the methyl radical (- CH_3). Main source is fish oil.

Emulsify. To mix two or more liquids that are normally immiscible. For example, to break oils into tiny droplets mixed with water (as in milk).

Enzyme. Substance (basically protein) that acts as a catalyst of biochemical reactions in the body. It promotes and accelerates biochemical reactions and is not consumed by the reaction itself.

EPA. See eicosapentaenoic acid.

Esophagus. Muscular tube through which food passes and that connects the pharynx to the stomach. Also called oesophagus.

Essential Amino Acids. Amino acids necessary for good health that cannot be synthesized by the body. They must be obtained from food sources.

Essential Fatty Acids (EFAs). Fatty acids necessary for good health that cannot be synthesized by the body. They must be obtained from dietary sources.

Essential Vitanutrients. Organic substances fundamental for health, necessary only in small quantities (micronutrient), that cannot be synthesized by the body's metabolism.

Estrogen. Primary female sex hormone produced in the ovaries and that generates the female characteristics.

Eukaryotic Cell. Cell of a living organism with complex structures enclosed within a membrane, in which the genetic material is contained in the nucleus.

Familial Hypercholesterolemia. Genetic disorder characterized by high levels of cholesterol in the blood, caused primarily by an inherited defect in LDL receptors.

Fat. Substance rich in saturated fatty acids, usually solid at room temperature.

Fatty Acids. Carboxylic acids formed of a long hydrocarbon chain linked to a carboxyl radical (- COOH). Fatty acids are the building blocks of lipids.

Fiber. Polysaccharide (long carbohydrate polymer) present in vegetables that is not digested by the body.

Fibrous Proteins. Insoluble proteins characterized by a rigid and long configuration, in the form of fibers.

Flavonoids. See bioflavonoids.

Flaxseed. Seed of a plant of the family Linaceae rich in omega-3 fatty acids, especially the essential alpha-linolenic acid (LNA), and in soluble fibers (lignans) with phytohormone properties.

Free Radical. Highly reactive molecular fragment seeking electrons from other molecules. It causes oxidative damage to the cells and tissues, and may lead to precocious aging, cardiovascular disease, and cancer.

Gallbladder. Small membrane-bound organ that aids mainly in fat digestion and concentrates bile produced by the liver.

Gamma-Linolenic Acid (GLA). Essential fatty acid (octadecatrienoic), of the omega-6 family, formed of an 18-carbon chain with three cis double bonds that occur in the carbons 6, 9, and 12, counting from the methyl radical (- CH_3). It is an isomer of alpha-linolenic acid.

Gene. A unique sequence of nucleotides that codify a polypeptide or an RNA chain. A molecular unit of heredity of a living organism.

Genetic Code. Correspondence between the sequence of nucleotides in the nucleic acid and the sequence of amino acids in a polypeptide (protein). The code defines how genetic material (DNA or mRNA sequences) is translated into proteins (amino acid sequences) by living cells.

Genome. The complete set of genetic instructions of an organism, or the entirety of an organism's hereditary information.

Genotype. Genetic makeup of a cell, an organism, or an individual.

GI. See Glycemic Index

GLA. See gamma-linolenic acid.

Gland. An organ or group of cells specialized in the synthesis of hormones for release in the blood stream or into cavities inside the body.

Glycation. Biochemical reaction of blood sugar with a protein or lipid molecule. Glycation damages tissue collagen and leads to cellular aging.

Glycemic Index (GI). Relative quantity or number that indicates the rate, or speed, at which glucose enters the blood stream after ingestion of foods that contain carbohydrates.

Glycemic Load (GL). Relative quantity or number obtained by multiplying the glycemic index (GI) of a carbohydrate food by the percent of carbohydrate in that food. It is an indicator of the effects of this food in the blood levels of glucose and insulin.

Glycogen. Polymer or macromolecule of glucose residues that serves as the secondary long-term energy storage in animal tissue.

Glycolysis. The biochemical metabolic pathway that converts glucose into pyruvate. The free energy released in this process is used to form the high-energy molecules of adenosine triphosphate (ATP).

Glicosylation. Enzymatic process that attaches carbohydrates (glycans) to proteins, lipids, or other organic molecules.

Globular Proteins. Proteins characterized by a compact globe-like or spherical configuration, such as hemoglobin. Also called spheroproteins.

Glucagon. A peptide hormone (made of 29 amino acids) secreted by the islets of Langerhans, in the pancreas, important mainly in the metabolism of glucose and lipids. Glucagon also regulates the rate of glucose production through lipolysis.

HDL. See high-density lipoprotein.

Health. State of total physical, mental, and social well-being.

Heart Attack. See myocardial infarction.

HGH. See human growth hormone.

High-Density Lipoprotein (HDL). Globular aggregate of cholesterol, lipids, and proteins, that removes excess cholesterol from the tissues and transport it, through the blood, back to the liver. It is popularly known as good cholesterol.

High-Quality Protein. Food rich in proteins, whose composition of essential amino acids is close to the ideal for utilization by the human body.

Homeostasis. Maintenance of a healthy and stable balance between body fluids and organ cells in a living organism.

Hormone. Chemical substance (peptide or steroid) released by an organ or tissue in the blood stream, in one part of the body, and which induces a physiological action (such as growth or metabolism) in another organ or tissue, remote from the secretion local. Hormones act as chemical messengers.

Human Growth Hormone (HGH). A peptide hormone, secreted by the pituitary gland, that stimulates anabolic processes, such as growth, cell reproduction and regeneration, and maintenance of body functions.

Hydrogenation. Industrial process that requires the presence of a catalyst, in which hydrogen is added to unsaturated vegetable oils, transforming them into vegetable fats solid at room temperature and more stable (such as margarine).

Hydrolysis. Chemical process in which a water molecule is used to break down a covalent chemical bond in a molecule, splitting it into two parts.

Hydrophilic Substance. Chemical substance of polar nature that can interact with water molecules. These substances are water-soluble.

Hydrophobic Substance. Chemical substance with non-polar properties that are soluble in non-polar solvents (as lipids), but not soluble in water.

Hydroxyl Group. Chemical radical or functional group (- OH) as part of an organic molecule.

Hypercholesterolemia. Presence of high levels of cholesterol in the blood, a risk factor for cardiovascular disease.

Hyperglycemia. Excessive levels of glucose circulating in the blood plasma.

Hyperinsulinism. Excessive production of the insulin hormone by the pancreas, as a result of excessive ingestion of high glycemic index (GI) carbohydrates.

Hypertension. See arterial hypertension.

Hypoglycemia. Abnormally diminished content of glucose in the blood.

IDL. See intermediate-density lipoprotein.

IGF-1. See insulin-like growth factor 1.

Ileocecal Sphincter. Circular muscle or anatomical ring valve that controls the opening and closure between the small intestine (ileum) and the large intestine.

Ileum. Final section of the small intestine, following the duodenum and jejunum.

Immunoglobulin. See antibody.

Incomplete Protein. Food rich in proteins, in which one or more of the essential amino acids are absent or present only in small quantities.

Insulin. Peptide hormone (composed of 51 amino acids) secreted by the islets of Langerhans in the pancreas to transport and process glucose in the blood.

Insulin-Like Growth Factor 1 (IGF-1). Hormonal substance similar in molecular structure to insulin, that acts together with the human growth hormone (HGH) to regulate body's metabolism and growth.

Insulin Resistance. Physiological inability of cells to effectively capture glucose under the action of the insulin hormone.

Intermediate-Density Lipoprotein (IDL). Globular aggregate of cholesterol, lipids, and proteins, that transports cholesterol and other lipids, through the blood, to the body's tissues. It has an intermediate density between LDL and VLDL.

Intestinal Villi. Small structures with many folds covered with tiny finger-like projections that protrude from the epithelial lining of the intestinal walls, similar to microscopic capillary structures, that greatly increase the internal area of the intestine walls for absorption of the nutrient molecules.

Jejunum. Middle section of the small intestine.

Ketogenesis. Synthesis of ketone bodies from acetyl-coenzyme A, in response to low glucose levels in the blood.

Ketone Bodies. Denomination given to three water-soluble compounds, namely acetone, acetoacetic acid, and beta-hydroxybutyric acid. They are produced from acetyl-CoA as by-products when fatty acids are broken down for energy in the liver and kidneys, in the absence of glucose. See also ketogenesis.

Ketose. (1) Sugar molecule in which its carbonyl group is a ketone (fructose is an example of a ketose). Ketoses can isomerize into an aldose when the carbonyl group is located at the end of the molecule. (2) Pathological metabolic condition characterized by excessive production of ketone molecules beyond the body's utilization capacity.

Krebs Cycle. See citric acid cycle.

LA. See linoleic acid.

LDL. See low-density lipoprotein.

Lecithin. Fatty nutrient that contains phospholipids, composed of fatty acids, glycerol, choline, and a phosphate group. It is a major component of the structure of cell membranes and other cellular components. Good food sources of lecithin include soy beans and egg yolk.

Leukocytes. White blood cells or cells of the immune system involved in defending the body against infectious disease and foreign elements.

Linoleic Acid (LA). Essential fatty acid (octadecadienoic), of the omega-6 family, formed of an 18-carbon chain with two cis double bonds that occur in the carbons 6, and 9, counting from the methyl radical ($- CH_3$). Saturating the n-6 double bond it is converted to oleic acid.

Linolenic Acid. See alpha-linolenic acid (LNA).

Linseed. See flaxseed.

Lipid. Any member of a broad group of naturally occurring molecules that include fatty acids, triglycerides, phospholipids, cholesterol, and sterols, which hydrophobic or lipophilic (not soluble in water) properties.

Lipogenesis. Process in which acetyl-coA is converted to fats, leading to body fat formation and accumulation.

Lipolysis. Process of breakdown of lipids for the body's metabolism.

Lipoprotein. Globular aggregate (or biochemical assembly) of molecules that consists of a non-polar lipid center involved by an amphiphilic layer of protein, phospholipids, and cholesterol, used to transport cholesterol and other lipids through the blood to the body's tissues.

LNA. See alpha-linolenic acid.

Low-Density Lipoprotein (LDL). Globular aggregate of cholesterol, lipids, and proteins that transports cholesterol and other lipids, through the blood, to the body's tissues. It is popularly known as bad cholesterol.

Lutein. Antioxidant substance that belongs to the naturally occurring carotenoids. It is a xanthophyll synthesized by plants. Good sources are green leafy vegetables, egg yolk, and animal fats.

Lycopene. Phytochemical pigment present in reddish colored fruits and vegetables (specially tomatoes), that strengthen the body's immune system and exert protective antioxidant action.

Lymphocyte. Some cells of the immune system.

Lysosome. Cell organelle delimited by a membrane in an eukaryotic cell, that contains hydrolytic enzymes.

Macronutrient. Substance needed in large quantities by the body, such as water, carbohydrates, proteins, and lipids.

Metabolic Fuel. Elementary molecule that can be oxidized (burned) through the body's metabolism, providing free energy to the body.

Metabolism. The whole set of chemical reactions necessary to sustain life in living organisms. Metabolism involves degradation reactions (catabolism), that liberate energy, and biosynthesis reactions (anabolism), that absorb energy.

Metabolite. Intermediate chemical reactant in metabolism or a product of metabolic reactions.

Methyl Group. Chemical radical or functional group (- CH_3) as part of an organic molecule.

Mitochondria. Cell organelles, enclosed by two membranes, found in the cytoplasm of most eukaryotic cells, in which metabolic reactions occur for chemical energy generation. They are tiny cellular power plants that include the oxidative reactions of the citric acid cycle (or Krebs cycle), fatty acid oxidation, and oxidative phosphorylation.

Molecule. Electrically neutral group of two or more atoms held together by covalent chemical bonds.

Monosaccharide. Single basic unit of sugars. Examples include glucose (dextrose), fructose (levulose), and galactose. They are the building blocks of disaccharides (such as sucrose) and polysaccharides (such as starch and cellulose).

Monounsaturated Fatty Acids (MUFAs). Fatty acids that contain only one double bond in their carbon atom chain. Most known is oleic acid, a healthy dietary component in olive oil.

MUFA. See monounsaturated fatty acids.

Mutation. Hereditary alteration in the genetic material (DNA or RNA sequence of a cell's genome) of a living organism.

Myocardial Infarction. Damage or death (infarction) of heart muscle tissue (myocardium) resulting from interruption (blockage) of blood and oxygen supply to the coronary arteries. Also known as heart attack.

Neurotransmitter. Chemical substance, released by a nervous cell, that transmits signals across the nervous system to alter the activity of another (target) nervous cell. It acts as a communication link between neurons (brain cells) and other cells of the nervous system. They are synthesized from simple precursors such as amino acids.

Nucleic Acids. Biological polymeric macromolecules of nucleotides, essential for life. Also called polynucleotides. Main ones are DNA (deoxyribonucleic acid) and RNA (ribonucleic acid).

Nucleus. Cell organelle, enclosed by a double membrane, found inside the eukaryotic cell, that contains most of its genetic material.

Nutrition. Science that studies the relations between the ingested food and the health and well-being of the human body.

Obesity. Abnormal accumulation of fats in the adipose tissues of the body.

Oil. Substance rich in polyunsaturated fatty acids, usually liquid at room temperature.

Oleic Acid. Monounsaturated omega-9 fatty acid (octadecenoic), formed of an 18-carbon chain with only one cis double bond that occurs right in the middle of the carbon chain. It is a healthy nutrient found primarily in olive oil, canola oil, peanuts, and macadamias.

Oligomer. Small chemical polymer that consists of a few monomer units bound together.

Oligosaccharide. Polymeric carbohydrate (saccharide) that contains a few residues (typically two to ten) of monosaccharides (simple sugars) bound together.

Omega-3 Fatty Acid. Denomination that refers to the chemical structure of unsaturated fatty acids, in which the first double bond occurs in the third carbon of the fatty acid carbon atom chain, counting from the methyl radical $(- CH_3)$.

Omega-6 Fatty Acid. Denomination that refers to the chemical structure of unsaturated fatty acids, in which the first double bond occurs in the sixth carbon of the fatty acid carbon atom chain, counting from the methyl radical $(- CH_3)$.

Omega-9 Fatty Acid. Denomination that refers to the chemical structure of unsaturated fatty acids, in which the first double bond occurs in the ninth carbon of the fatty acid carbon atom chain, counting from the methyl radical $(- CH_3)$.

Organelle. Differentiated subunit structure inside an eukaryotic cell that has a specific function, such as mitochondria, vacuoles, ribosomes, lysosomes, or nucleus.

Orthomolecular Medicine. Preservation of good health and treatment of physical and mental disorders through the use of substances or orthomolecular nutrients normally present in the body.

Orthomolecular Substance. Substance, or vitanutrient, normally present in the human body, that is necessary for life and good health.

Osmosis. Net movement of solvent molecules through a partially permeable membrane (permeable to the solvent, but not the solute), into a region of higher solute concentration.

Oxidizing Agent. Substance that removes electrons from another reactant in a redox chemical reaction. The oxidizing agent is reduced by receiving the electron and the other reactant is oxidized by having its electron removed. Oxygen is a main oxidizing agent.

Oxidoreductase. Chemical enzyme that catalyzes a reduction-oxidation (redox) reaction, that is, the transfer of electrons from the reductant (electron donor) to the oxidant (electron acceptor).

Partially-Hydrogenated Vegetable Oil. Vegetable oil altered by industrial chemical processes, in which hydrogen is added to some double bonds between carbon atoms to saturate some fatty acid molecules, leaving some double bonds in the stereoisomeric forms cis and trans.

Peptidase. Enzyme that promotes proteolysis, that is, protein catabolism by hydrolysis of the peptide (amino acid chain) bonds. It is also called protease or proteinase.

Peptide. Short chemical polymer of amino acid monomers linked by peptide bonds. They constitute the basic structure units of proteins.

Peptide Bond. Covalent chemical bond formed between the amino group of an amino acid and the carboxyl group of another, joining residues of amino acids into a polypeptide.

Peptide Group. Chemical planar group in the form - CO - NH -, which includes a covalent peptide bond between residues of amino acids in a polypeptide.

Peristalsis. Sequence of contraction and relaxation movements of the smooth muscles of the gastrointestinal tract, that slowly moves the ingested (and digested) food throughout the gastrointestinal tract.

PG. See prostaglandin.

pH. Numerical quantity used in chemistry that specifies the acidity or basicity of an aqueous solution. It is defined as the negative logarithm of the hydrogen ion concentration (- $\log [H^+]$) in a solution. A neutral aqueous solution has pH = 7; acid solutions, pH < 7; and alkaline solutions, pH > 7. Blood is normally a slightly alkaline fluid with a pH around 7.4.

Phenols. Chemical substances that have an hydroxyl (- OH) group (as in alcohols) attached to an aromatic benzenoid (phenyl) carbon ring.

Phospholipids. A class of fatty acids that contain the phosphorus element in its molecule. They are a major component of all cell membranes. The most known example is lecithin.

Photo-respiration. A process in plant metabolism that involves carbon dioxide consumption and oxygen production. Dissipation of photosynthesis products.

Photosynthesis. Reduction of carbon dioxide to carbohydrates, in plants and bacteria, promoted by light energy and with liberation of oxygen.

Phytochemicals. Chemical substances present naturally in plants that are responsible for their color and organoleptic properties (from the Greek *phuton*, which means *plant*).

Polymer. A large molecule (macromolecule) composed of many repeating smaller subunits (monomers) structurally bound to one another. They may be linearly structured or ramified.

Polypeptide. Short polymer that consists of amino acid monomers (peptides) linked by peptide bonds.

Polyphenols. Phytochemical organic substances found in many vegetables and fruits that exert protective antioxidant action in the body. They are composed of many (*poly*) multiples of *phenol* structure units.

Polysaccharide. Polymeric carbohydrate that consists of a long chain of monosaccharide (single sugar) monomers joined together by glycosidic bonds. Also known as glycan.

Polyunsaturated Fat. See polyunsaturated fatty acids (PUFAs).

Polyunsaturated Fatty Acids (PUFAs). Fatty acids that contain more than one double bond in their carbon atom chain.

Portal Vein. Hepatic vein that conducts the blood from the stomach, intestine, pancreas, and gallbladder into the liver, where it divides into a capillary system (hepatic sinusoids).

Precursor. Compound that participates in a chemical reaction to produce another substance or that precedes another in a metabolic pathway.

Primrose Oil. Oil from the seeds of a flowering plant known as evening-primrose. It is rich in linoleic acid (LA) and gamma-linolenic acid (GLA).

Proenzyme. An inactive enzyme precursor. Also known as zymogen.

Prostaglandins. Substances produced enzymatically from fatty acids in many places throughout the body that exert actions similar to hormones (messenger molecules), but of short duration and reach. They play important functions in the control and regulation of many cellular activities. Chemically they contain 20 carbon atoms that include a 5-carbon ring.

Protease. See peptidase.

Proteins. Polymeric macromolecules that consist of one or more polypeptide chains constituted of amino acids. They play myriads of important functions in the body.

Ptyalin. Salivary enzyme that initiates the breakdown of carbohydrates from food.

PUFA. See polyunsaturated fatty acids.

Pyloric Sphincter. Circular muscle or anatomical ring valve that controls the opening and closure between the stomach and the small intestine (ileum).

Receptor. A protein molecule, most often present on the surface of a cell, that specifically binds to a hormone, neurotransmitter, or another ligand, and that signals the cell to perform some specific biological activity.

Redox Reaction. Reduction-oxidation chemical reaction that involves an oxidizing substance (free radical, seeking electrons) and a reducing substance (antioxidant, electron donor). Antioxidants are used to neutralize the cell damaging action of free radicals.

Reduction Agent. Substance that provides electrons and becomes oxidized in a redox reaction.

Residue. Term used in chemistry for the monomeric unit of a polymer.

Resveratrol. A phenol substance produced naturally by several plants and found in the skin and seeds of red grapes (also in red wine) and other fruits and vegetables. Studies indicate that it may have anti-aging, anticancer, anti-inflammatory, and blood-sugar lowering effects, as well as other beneficial cardiovascular effects.

Ribonucleic Acid (RNA). Polymeric macromolecule of ribonucleotides. The sequence of nucleotides allows RNA to encode genetic information. The main forms of RNA include the messenger RNA (mRNA), the transfer RNA (tRNA), and the ribosomal RNA (rRNA).

RNA. See ribonucleic acid.

Saccharide. See carbohydrate.

Salivary Amylase. See ptyalin.

Saturated Fat. See saturated fatty acids (SFAs).

Saturated Fatty Acids (SFAs). Fatty acids with no double bonds, but only single bonds, in their carbon atom chain.

Somatostatin. Peptide hormone produced by the islets of Langerhans, in the pancreas, that regulates the endocrine system and acts to inhibit the release of other hormones, including insulin and the human growth hormone.

Sphincter. Circular muscle or anatomical ring valve that controls the opening and closure of a natural body passage or orifice.

Starch. Carbohydrate (polysaccharide) that consists of polymers (linear or ramified) of glucose units joined together by glycosidic bonds. It constitutes the main energy reserve in plants and vegetables. Its main components are amylopectin and amylose. Also called amylum.

Stereoisomers. Isomeric molecules that have the same molecular formula and sequence of bond connections between the constituent atoms, but differ in the 3D spatial orientation of their atoms.

Steroids. Natural lipids that contains four cycloalkane carbon rings joined to each other. Many steroids are hormones derived from cholesterol.

Sterols. Organic substances derived from steroids, also known as steroid alcohols. Sterols of plants are called phytosterols.

Stroke. Rapid loss of brain functions due to disturbances in the blood supply to the brain, which can result from lack of blood flow (schemia) caused by blockage (thrombosis, arterial embolism), or leakage of blood (hemorrhage).

Substrate. Reactant molecule in an enzymatic chemical reaction.

Sucrose. A disaccharide commonly known as table sugar and sometimes called saccharose. It is normally obtained from sugar cane, beetroots, or honey. During digestion it is broken into the monosaccharides glucose and fructose.

Sugar. Generalised name for a class of sweet-flavored carbohydrates. Simple sugars, called monosaccharides, include glucose, fructose, and galactose. Disaccharides include sucrose (table sugar), maltose, and lactose.

Synapse. Nervous system structure that permits a neuron (brain cell) to pass an electrical or chemical signal to another cell (neural or otherwise).

Testosterone. Steroid hormone from the androgen group or male sexual hormone.

Thermodynamics. Science that studies the relations between the various forms of energy.

Thermogenesis. Energy generation process for body heat.

Trace-Mineral. Mineral substance used by the body in small quantities.

Trans Fat. Artificial antinutrient, harmful to the body and its metabolism, generated in the industrial process of partial hydrogenation of vegetable oils.

Transgene. Non-native segment of DNA, containing a gene sequence, that has been introduced into a different organism.

Triacylglycerols. See triglycerides.

Tricarboxylic Acid Cycle (TCA). See citric acid cycle.

Triglycerides. Lipids in which three fatty acid molecules are chemically bound to a glycerol molecule. Also known as triacylglycerols. They are the form in which fatty acids are stored in the tissues of animals and plants.

Type 1 Diabetes. See diabetes mellitus type 1

Type 2 Diabetes. See diabetes mellitus type 2.

Ubiquinone. See coenzyme Q_{10} .

UFA. See unsaturated fatty acids.

Unsaturated Fat. See unsaturated fatty acids (UFAs).

Unsaturated Fatty Acids (UFAs). Fatty acids that contain one or more double bonds in their carbon atom chain.

Vacuole. Membrane-bound intracellular organelle which is filled with water containing inorganic and organic molecules, including enzymes.

Very-Low Density Lipoprotein (VLDL). Globular aggregate of cholesterol, lipids, and proteins, that transports cholesterol and other lipids, through the blood, to the body's tissues. It has an intermediate density between chylomicron and IDL, and transports mainly triglycerides.

Villus. See intestinal villi.

Vitamin. Organic compound, usually essential, that acts in the body mainly to control and regulate the metabolic processes. Each one of the many vitamins plays a decisive role in vital processes in cells and tissues.

Vitanutrient. Organic substance, fundamental for the body's health and well-being, that is necessary only in small quantities (micronutrient).

VLDL. See very-low density lipoprotein.

Zeaxanthin. A common carotenoid alcohol, present in many vegetables, that exert protective antioxidant action to the body's cells and tissues. It is one of the two primary xanthophyll carotenoids present in the retina of the eye. It is an isomer of lutein.

BIBLIOGRAPHY

1. Atkins, Robert C. **Dr. Atkins' age-defying diet.** New York: St. Martins Press, 2001.

2. Atkins, Robert C. **Dr. Atkins' new carbohydrate gram counter.** New York: M. Evans and Company, 1996.

3. Atkins, Robert C. **Dr. Atkins' new diet cookbook.** New York: M. Evans and Company Pub., 1997.

4. Atkins, Robert C. **Dr. Atkins' new diet revolution** (revised and updated). New York: Avon Books, 1999.

5. Ballentine, Rudolph. **Diet and nutrition: a holistic approach.** Honesdale, PA, The Himalayan Institute Press, 2007.

6. Barilla, Jean (Editor). **The nutrition superbook. Volume 1: the anti-oxidants.** Connecticut: Keats Publishing Inc., 1996.

7. Barilla, Jean (Editor). **The nutrition superbook. Volume 2: the good fats and oils.** Connecticut: Keats Publishing Inc., 1996.

8. Bender, David A. **Introduction to nutrition and metabolism.** New York: Taylor & Francis, Third Edition, 2002.

9. Boyle Marie A.; Zyla, Gail. **Personal nutrition.** Minneapolis: West Pub. Co., 1996.

10. Brand-Miller, Jennie; Wolever, Thomas M. S.; Colagiuri, Stephen; Foster-Powell, Kaye. **The glucose revolution: the authoritative guide to the glycemic index.** Marlowe and Co. Publishers, 1999.

11. Brody, Tom. **Nutritional biochemistry.** New York: Academic Press, Second Edition, 1999.

12. Carper, Jean. **Food: your miracle medicine.** New York: HarperCollins Publishers Inc., 1998.

13. Carper, Jean. **Miracle cures.** New York: HarperCollins Publishers Inc., 1998.

14. Carper, Jean. **Stop aging now.** New York: HarperCollins Publishers Inc., 1996.

15. Carper, Jean. **The miracle heart.** New York: HarperCollins Publishers Inc., 2000.

16. Carper, Jean. **Your miracle brain.** Quill Publishing, 2002.

17. Cody; Mildred M. **Safe food for you and your family.** Minneapolis: The American Dietetic Association, Chronimed Publishing, 1996.

18. Colpo, Anthony. **The great cholesterol con.** Lulu, USA, Second Edition, 2006.

19. Consumer Guide Editors, with the Nutrient Analysis Center. **The complete food count guide.** Illinois: Chicago Center for Clinical Research, Lincolnwood Publications, Ltd., 1996.

20. Cordain, Loren. **The Paleo diet.** New Jersey: John Wiley & Sons, Inc., 2011.

21. Crayon, Robert. **Nutrition made simple.** New York: M. Evans and Company Inc., 1994.

22. Davis, William. **Wheat belly.** New York: Rodale Inc., 2011.

23. Dunne, Lavon, J. **Nutrition almanac.** Fifth Edition, McGraw-Hill Professional Publishing, 2001.

24. Duyff, Roberta Larson. **American dietetic association complete food and nutrition guide.** Hoboken, New Jersey: John Wiley & Sons, Third Edition, 2006.

25. Eades, Michael R.; Eades, Mary Dan; Eades, Mary. **The protein power lifeplan.** Warner Books, 2001.

26. Enig, Mary G. **Know your fats: the complete primer for understanding the nutrition of fats, oils and cholesterol.** Bethesda Press, 2000.

27. Erickson, Martha A. **Eat for the Health of It.** Philadelphia, Starburst Publishers, Lancaster, 1997.

28. Gershoff, Stanley N.; Whitney, Catherine; and the Editorial Advisory Board of the Tufts University Health & Nutrition Letter, **The Tufts University guide to total nutrition.** New York: Harper Perennial, Second Edition, 1996.

29. Gittleman, Ann Louise. **Eat fat, lose weight.** Illinois: Keats Publishing, 1999.

30. Gittleman, Ann Louise. **The fat flush plan.** McGraw-Hill Professional Publishing, 2001.

31. Graveline, Duane. **Lipitor: thief of memory.** www.spacedoc.net, 2006.

32. Groff, James L.; Gropper, Sareen S. **Advanced nutrition and human metabolism.** Wadsworth Publishing, Third Edition, 1999.

33. Gropper, Sareen S.; Smith, Jack L. **Advanced nutrition and human metabolism.** Belmont, CA: Wadsworth Publishing, 2008.

34. Hendler, Sheldon S.; Rorvik, David. **PDR for nutritional suplements.** First Edition, Medical Economics Company, 2001.

35. Kendrick, Malcolm. **The great cholesterol con.** London, England: John Blake Publishing, 2007.

36. Kirschmann, Gayla J. **Nutrition almanac.** Fourth Edition, McGraw-Hill, 1996.

37. Krummel Debra A.; Kris-Etherton Penny M. (Editors). **Nutrition in**

women's health. Gaithersburg, MD: Aspen Publisher's, 1996.

38. Lehninger, Albert L.; Nelson, David L.; Cox, Michael M. **Principles of biochemistry.** Third Edition, New York: Worth Publishing Inc., 2000.

39. Montgomery, Rex; Conway, Thomas W.; Spector, Arthur A. **Biochemistry: a case oriented approach.** Fifth Edition, The C. V. Mosby Company, 1994.

40. Natow, Annette B.; Heslin, Jo-Ann. **The fat counter.** The revised and updated 4th Edition. New York: Pocket Books, 1998.

41. Netzer, Corinne T. **The complete book of food counts.** Fifth Edition, New York: Dell Publishing Co., 2000.

42. Page, Helen Cassidy; Schroeder, John Speer; Dickson, Tara C. **The Stanford life plan for a healthy heart.** San Francisco, CA: Chronicle Books, 1996.

43. Pauling, Linus C. **How to live longer and feel better.** Reissue Edition, Avon Publishing, 1996.

44. Passwater, Richard A. **All about antioxidants.** McGraw-Hill, 1998.

45. Passwater, Richard A. **The antioxidants.** McGraw-Hill, 1997.

46. Phyllis, A.; Balch, C. N. C.; James, F.; Balch, M. D. **Prescription for nutritional healing.** Avery Penguin Putman Pub., 2000.

47. Pressman, Alan H.; Buff, Sheila. **Glutathione: the ultimate antioxidant.** St. Martin Press, 1998.

48. Ravnskov, Uffe. **Fat and cholesterol are good for you.** GB Pub., Sweden, 2009.

49. Rinzler, Carol Ann. **Nutrition for dummies.** Chicago: IDG Books Worldwide, 1997.

50. Roizen, Michael F.; La Puma, John. **The real age diet.** New York: HarperCollins Publishers Inc., 2001.

51. Roizen, Michael F.; Oz, Mehmet C. **You: the owner´s manual.** New York: Harper Collins Publishers, 2005; Updated and expanded edition, 2008.

52. Roizen, Michael F.; Oz, Mehmet C. **You: on a diet.** New York: Free Press, Simon and Schuster Inc., 2006.

53. Roizen, Michael F.; Oz, Mehmet C. **You: staying young.** New York: Free Press, Simon and Schuster Inc., 2007.

54. Roizen, Michael F.; Oz, Mehmet C. **You: losing weight.** New York: Free Press, Simon and Schuster Inc., 2011.

55. Rowan, Robert. **Control high blood pressure without drugs.** New York: Simon and Schuster Inc., 2001.

56. Sahelion, Ray; Challem, Jack. **All about coenzime Q_{10} (frequently asked questions).** New York: Avery Penguin Putman Pub., 1999.

57. Shabert, Judy; Erlich, Nancy. **The ultimate nutrient: glutamine.** New York: Avery Pub., 1994.

58. Sifton, David W. (Editor). **The PDR family guide to nutrition and health.** New Jersey: Medical Economics, 1995.

59. Sisson, Mark. **The primal blueprint.** Malibu, CA: Primal Nutrition Inc., 2009.

60. Sinatra, Stephen T.; Sinatra, Jan DeMarco. **L-carnitine and the heart.** McGraw-Hill, 1999.

61. Sinatra, Stephen T. **The coenzime Q10 phenomenon: the breakthrough nutrient that helps combat heart disease, cancer, aging and more.** Mc-Graw Hill, 1998.

62. Sizer, Francis; Whitney, Ellie. **Nutrition: concepts and controversies.** Belmont, CA: The Thomson Corp., 2007.

63. Smolin, Lori A.; Grosvenor, Mary B. **Nutrition: science and applications.** Wiley Text Books, Fifth Edition, 2010.

64. Sonberg, Lynn. **The complete nutrition counter.** Berkley Pub. Group, 1993.

65. Stryer, Lubert. **Biochemistry.** W. H. Freeman Publishers, 1995.

66. Thompson, Jean A. (Editor). **The essential guide to nutrition and the foods we eat.** New York: Harper Collins Pub., 1999.

67. Turner, Elaine; Ross, Don; Insel, Paul. **Nutrition.** Jones & Bartlett Publishers, Second Edition, 2004.

68. Trugo, Luiz; Finglas, Paul; Caballero, Benjamin. **Encyclopedia of food sciences and nutrition.** (Ten-volume set). New York: Academic Press, Second Edition, 2003.

69. Voet, Donald; Voet, Judith C.; Pratt, Charlotte W. **Fundamentals of biochemistry.** John Wiley & Sons Inc., 1999.

70. Wade, Jr., L. G. **Organic chemistry.** Fourth Edition, Prentice Hall, 1998.

71. Weil, Andrew; Daley, Rosie. **The healthy kitchen.** New York: Random House Inc., 2002.

72. Weil, Andrew. **Eating well for optimum health.** New York: HarperCollins Publisher Inc., 2001.

73. Weil, Andrew. **Eight weeks to optimum health.** New York: Random House, 1998.

74. Weil, Andrew. **Spontaneous healing.** New York: Random House Inc., 1996.

75. Wennik, Roberta Schwartz. **Beyond food labels: eating healthy with the % daily values.** New York: Berkley Pub. Group, 1996.

76. Whitney, Eleanor Noss; Rolfes, Sharon Rady. **Understanding nutrition.** Belmont, CA: Wadsworth Publishing, 2007.

77. Willet, Walter C.; Skerrett, P. J. **Eat, drink and be healthy: the Harvard medical school guide to healthy eating.** New York: Simon and Schuster, 2005.

78. Wiseman, Gerald. **Nutrition and health.** New York: Taylor & Francis, 2002.

INDEX

ABOUT THE AUTHOR

JOSE AUGUSTO BITTENCOURT (born June 08, 1947, in Araguari, Minas Gerais, Brazil) is a physicist who for more than 40 years has been actively researching Plasma Physics, Space Science, and Aeronomy. More recently, in the past 15 years, he has also done extensive research on Nutritional Biochemistry.

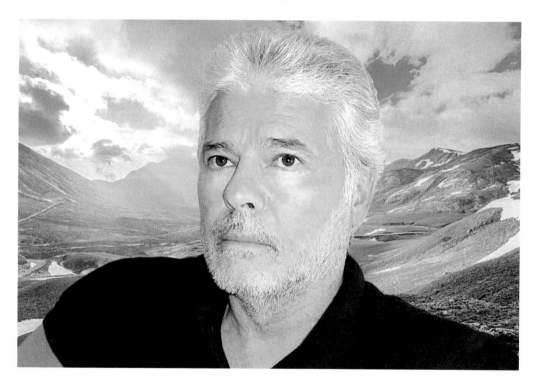

He received his Ph.D. degree in Physics from the University of Texas at Dallas – UTD (USA) in 1975. Since then he has been a Research Scientist and Graduate-level Professor at the National Institute for Space Research – INPE (Sao Jose dos Campos, Sao Paulo, Brazil) and has served many scientific organizations. He is also graduated (B.Sc.) in Chemical Engineering (1970) from the Federal University of Minas Gerais - UFMG (Belo Horizonte, Brazil) and received a Master of Sciences (M.Sc.) degree in Space Science from the National Institute for Space Research - INPE in 1972.

His research interests include basic and applied plasma physics, ionospheric and magnetospheric plasmas, upper atmosphere physics, aeronomy, plasma dynamical processes, and computer simulation of plasma phenomena both in the laboratory and in space.

He has published more than 200 papers and scientific articles [1] in well-known international research journals such as *Journal of Geophysical Research (Space Science), Geophysical Research Letters, Journal of Atmospheric and Solar-Terrestrial Physics, Planetary and Space Sciences, Advances in Space Research, Plasma Physics and Controlled Fusion, Applied Physics Letters,* and *Geophysical Journal International Annales Geophysicae.*

He is also author of the book *Fundamentals of Plasma Physics* (704p., Third Edition, 2004, Hardcover; 2010, Paperback) published by Springer (USA).

Since 1975 he has taught graduate-level courses at INPE on plasma physics, electrodynamics, propagation of electromagnetic waves, thermodynamics, kinetic theory, quantum mechanics, ionospheric physics, and dynamics of the upper atmosphere. He has been also a graduate-level Conference Professor on plasma physics at the Aeronautics Institute of Technology - ITA (Sao Jose dos Campos) and, since 2004, a research collaborator at the University of Paraiba Valley - UNIVAP (Sao Jose dos Campos).

At INPE he was Head of the graduate courses on Space Science and on Plasma Physics, and also Head of the Aeronomy Department. He has been also an official member of the Commission H (Waves in Plasmas) of the International Union of Radio Science - URSI and Associate Editor of the *Brazilian Journal of Geophysics*, in the field of Aeronomy. Since 1989 he is a Research Fellowship member of the National Council for Scientific and Technological Development – CNPq (Brazil).

An especial interest has been dedicated to the study of Nutritional Science and the biochemical effects of the many nutrients in the human body. This research resulted in the books *Nutricao e Saude: Como Fazer Escolhas Sensatas em Dieta e Nutricao* (Portuguese, Sixth Edition, 2018) and *The Power of Carbohydrates, Proteins, and Lipids* (Fourth Edition, 2018), both printed by *CreateSpace*, an *Amazon.com* Company (USA).

[1] https://www.researchgate.net/profile/J_Bittencourt

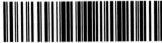

Made in the USA
Middletown, DE
16 January 2019